Medicines Management in Adult Nursing

Series Editors: Shirley Bach and Mooi Standing

Transforming Nursing Practice series

Transforming Nursing Practice links theory with practice, in the context of the skills and knowledge needed by student nurses to be fit for future healthcare delivery. Each book has been designed to help students meet the requirements of the NMC Standards of Education, Essential Skills Clusters and other relevant competencies. They are accessible and challenging, and provide regular opportunities for active and reflective learning. Each book will ensure that students learn the central importance of thinking critically about nursing.

Series editors:

Dr Shirley Bach, Head of the School of Nursing and Midwifery at the University of Brighton and Dr Mooi Standing, Principal Lecturer/Quality Lead in the Department of Nursing and Applied Clinical Studies, Canterbury Christ Church University.

Titles in the series:

To order, contact our distributor: BEBC Distribution, Albion Close, Parkstone, Poole, BH12 3LL. Telephone 0845 230 9000, email: **learningmatters@bebc.co.uk**. You can also find more information on each of these titles and our other learning resources at **www.learningmatters.co.uk**. Many of these titles are also available in various ebook formats. Please visit our website for more information.

Medicines Management in Adult Nursing

Elizabeth Lawson and Dawn L Hennefer

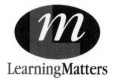
LearningMatters

First published in 2010 by Learning Matters Ltd

British Library Cataloguing in Publication Data
A CIP record for this book is available from the British Library

ISBN: 978 1 84445 842 4

This book is also available in the following ebook formats:

Adobe ebook: 978 1 84445 844 8
EPUB ebook: 978 1 84445 843 1
Kindle: 978 0 85725 046 9

2530402X

Cover design by Toucan Design
Project Management by Diana Chambers
Typeset by Kelly Gray
Printed and bound in Great Britain by TJ International Ltd, Padstow, Cornwall

Learning Matters Ltd
33 Southernhay East
Exeter EX1 1NX
Tel: 01392 215560
E-mail: info@learningmatters.co.uk
www.learningmatters.co.uk

FSC
Mixed Sources
Product group from well-managed forests and other controlled sources
Cert no. SGS-COC-2482
www.fsc.org
© 1996 Forest Stewardship Council

Contents

Foreword

The management and administration of medicines is a key aspect of nursing practice and is one of the most common therapeutic interventions in healthcare. Administering medications is often regarded as a ritualistic nursing behaviour associated with the drugs round, a trolley and keys signifying its status and mystical importance. However, as we know, it is far more than this and becoming more so as the underpinning knowledge of domains of arithmetic, law, ethics, pharmacology, evidence-based practice and working in different settings of care play an increasingly significant role in this area of nursing practice. Since 2003 the responsibilities of medicines management by nurses have increased with the introduction of the nursing formulary and nurse prescribing or the use of local prescribing protocols. This text is not intended to support such developed roles as they require additional training, but these developments are indicative of the range of responsibilities now associated with nursing care.

This text provides the key to unlocking the fundamental mysteries of medicines management as a preparation for student nurses and would also be suitable for qualified staff wishing to review their knowledge. It is thorough and clearly written, beginning with a review of your arithmetical skills which can then send you off on a path to deeper understanding of the law and ethical considerations, the complexities of pharmacological knowledge, establishing good practice and learning the techniques of medication administration.

The authors have taken a wider view of medicines management to include communication issues, working with other professionals and working in different settings of care – for example, child health and community settings. There is a focus on patients as partners and issues around adherence and culture explored. In the final chapter the evidence for practising is explored within a model that considers evidence as central and influenced by patient preference, critical appraisal and professional judgements. There are many activities and examples to help you embed the knowledge into your practice. By the end of this text you will not only know how – you will also know why, when and where!

Shirley Bach
Series Editor

Acknowledgements

The authors and publisher would like to thank the following for permission to reproduce copyright material:

The Information Services Department of the Library of the Health Sciences-Chicago, University of Illinois at Chicago for permission to reprint the 'Levels of Evidence Pyramid' from *Evidence-Based Practice in the Health Sciences: Evidence-Based Nursing Tutorial*, online tutorial at http://ebp.lib.uic.edu/nursing/?q=node/12.

Every effort has been made to trace all copyright holders within the book, but if any have been inadvertently overlooked the publisher will be pleased to make the necessary arrangements at the first opportunity.

About the authors

Dawn Gawthorpe is a senior lecturer in adult nursing at the School of Nursing and Midwifery at the University of Salford and teaches across pre-registration programmes. She was until recently the programme lead for the Diploma HE/RN (Adult Nursing) programme, and is the Exams and Assessment lead for the school of Nursing and Midwifery. Dawn has a special interest in neurosurgery, medical law and ethics.

Dawn L Hennefer is a Registered nurse and lecturer in Adult Nursing at the University of Salford with a background in teaching physiology, pharmacology and medicines management within clinical skills. She is currently Programme Leader for the Diploma of Higher Education/BSc Ordinary Degree (RN Adult) programme and co-leads Clinical Skills within pre-registration education across both degree and diploma programmes.

Elizabeth Lawson is a lecturer in the School of Nursing and Midwifery at the University of Salford with a clinical background mainly in child health nursing. She teaches physiology, pharmacology and pathology to undergraduate and postgraduate healthcare professionals.

Melanie Stephens is a lecturer in adult nursing at the University of Salford. Melanie has a background in Tissue viability, Inter-professional education and practice and Medical ethics and law.

Sarah Ratcliffe is a lecturer in Adult Nursing at the University of Salford. She is a Registered nurse with a background in Neuroscience nursing. Sarah has taught evidence-based practice and research to both undergraduate and post-qualifying nursing students.

Suzanne Waugh is Learning Skills tutor at the University of Salford. Her background is in both Archaeology and Psychology, and she currently runs the University's study skills programme. Suzanne is also a qualified adult numeracy teacher, and is developing numeracy provision for student nurses.

Introduction

Who is this book for?

This book explores the fundamental principles of medicines management in adult nursing, and is primarily for adult nursing students, explaining the potential risks in managing medicines so that patient safety can be maintained. It is aimed at students of adult nursing in order to inform their clinical practice, but as nurses work in a multi-disciplinary team the material covered is relevant to all health professionals. Other books in this series deal specifically with the issues of medicines management in other fields of practice. Medicines management is relevant wherever drugs are used in the therapeutic management of patients, so the book is for those working in hospitals, in the community, and in all other settings. Nurses are required to inform patients about their medicines in an accurate and helpful way, to have good numerical ability and to have excellent communication and interpersonal skills. The chapters of this book simplify some of the more complex issues in these requirements.

Book structure

Chapter 1, Drug calculations, introduces the numerical skills used within medicines management. Initially the reader can review number value and the four mathematical functions (addition, subtraction, multiplication and division). The conversion of units of measurement for medicines is covered, as well as the application of number, functions and units in drug calculation formulae.

Chapter 2, The law governing medicines, focuses on the legal aspects of medicines management, both to ensure you as the student nurse are protected by addressing accountability and duty of care, but also to ensure that the patient is protected from harm. Key legislation and the different categories of law are explored; although the book is adult focused, there may be occasions when adult nursing students engage professionally with children, so the ability to consent as a minor is included.

Chapter 3, Ethical frameworks, discusses ethical dilemmas in practice related to medicines management. The ethical and moral obligations of the student nurse are discussed, and there follows an account of ethical theories and ethical tenets, which are subsequently applied to practice examples and activities.

Chapter 4, Pharmacology, concentrates on how drugs work to be of therapeutic benefit to the patient. Routes of administration, the action of the medicine and side effects are covered, and the chapter also aims to provide an understanding of how age, gender, co-existing disease and other factors can impact on the patient.

Chapter 5, Medicines administration, familiarises the adult nursing student with the relevant NMC standards, in particular standard 8, and its practical application within medicines management. It includes practical elements of administering medicines to inform the student and prevent medication errors.

Chapter 6, Partnership working, deals with a team approach with patient centrality in medicine management. The adult nursing student can play a valuable role within the team approach, but this requires an understanding of the roles of both professional and non-professional healthcare workers. Nurse prescribing and the use of complementary and alternative therapies are discussed within this chapter.

Chapter 7, Evidence-based practice, examines the skills required for clinical decision making and evidence-based practice in medicines management to maintain patient safety. The chapter suggests sources of evidence available and how this evidence can be found, appraised and applied. Within this chapter activities are provided for the student to engage in, using high-quality information to inform their practice and develop their awareness of how evidence is positioned within a hierarchy framework.

Requirements for the NMC Standards for Pre-registration Nursing Education and Essential Skills Clusters

The Nursing and Midwifery Council (NMC) has established standards of competence to be met by applicants to different parts of the register, and these are the standards it considers necessary for safe and effective practice. In addition to the competencies, the NMC has set out specific skills that nursing students must be able to perform at various points of an education programme. These are known as Essential Skills Clusters (ESCs). This book is structured so that it will help you to understand and meet the competencies and ESCs required for entry to the NMC register. In particular, it addresses and is structured around the medicines management ESC. The relevant competencies and ESCs are presented at the start of each chapter so that you can clearly see which ones the chapter addresses. There are *generic standards* that all nursing students, irrespective of their field, must achieve and *field-specific standards* relating to each field of nursing, i.e. mental health, children, learning disability and adult nursing. Most chapters have generic standards, and occasionally field-specific standards are listed.

This book includes the latest draft standards for 2010 onwards, taken from *Standards for pre-registration nursing education: Draft for consultation* (NMC, January 2010). For links to the pre-2010 standards, please visit the website for the book at www.learningmatters.co.uk/nursing. This website will also list any amendments to the standards when the final version is published in October 2010.

Learning features

Activities

Throughout the book you will find activities in the text that will help you to make sense of, and learn about, the material being presented by the authors.

Some activities ask you to reflect on aspects of practice, or your experience of it, or the people or situations you encounter. *Reflection* is an essential skill in nursing, and it helps you to understand the world around you and often to identify how things might be improved. Other activities will help you develop key skills such as your ability to *think critically* about a topic in order to challenge received wisdom, or your ability to *research a topic and find appropriate information and evidence*, and to be able to make decisions using that evidence in situations that are often difficult and time-pressured. Finally, communication and working as part of a team are core to all nursing practice, and some activities will ask you to carry out *team work activities* or think about your *communication skills* to help develop these.

All the activities require you to take a break from reading the text, think through the issues presented and carry out some independent study, possibly using the internet. Where appropriate, there are sample answers presented at the end of each chapter, and these will help you to understand more fully your own reflections and independent study. Remember, academic study will always require independent work; attending lectures will never be enough to be successful on your programme, and these activities will help to deepen your knowledge and understanding of the issues under scrutiny and give you practice at working on your own.

You might want to think about completing these activities as part of your personal development plan (PDP) or portfolio. After completing the activity, write it up in your PDP or portfolio in a section devoted to that particular skill, then look back over time to see how far you are developing. You can also do more of the activities for a key skill that you have identified a weakness in, which will help build your skill and confidence in this area.

Chapter 1

Drug calculations

Suzanne Waugh

Draft NMC Standards for Pre-registration Nursing Education

This chapter will address the following draft competencies:

Domain: Nursing practice and decision making

Generic competencies:

4. All nurses must know the limitations and known hazards in the use of a range of technical nursing skills, activities, interventions, treatments, medical devices and equipment. This must include safe application and evaluation of the outcome in a variety of care settings, including complex, technical, diverse environments, to provide effective person centred care for people of all ages and backgrounds. Interventions will include safe medicines management, wound management, pain relief, and infection prevention and control. The nurse must report any concerns through appropriate channels and modify the plan of care to maintain safe practice.

Field specific competencies:

1.1. Adult nurses must safely use a range of diagnostic and clinical skills, complemented by existing and developing technology, to assess the nursing care of individuals undergoing therapeutic or clinical interventions.

Draft Essential Skills Clusters

This chapter will address the following draft ESCs:

Cluster: Medicines management

33. People can trust the newly registered graduate nurse to correctly and safely undertake medicines calculations.

By the first progression point:

i.   Is competent in basic medicines calculations.

By entry to the register:

ii. Accurately calculates medicines and ensures those responsible to the nurse are competent to do the same.

Chapter aims

After reading this chapter, you will be able to:

- use the 'four rules' (addition, subtraction, multiplication and division) to carry out a range of calculations, including with decimals;
- convert between different SI units;
- calculate how many tablets or how much liquid is needed to fill a prescription;
- use drug calculation formulae to answer more complex questions about the amount of a drug required and the number of drops per minute needed for intravenous fluids.

Introduction

Joanne Evans, a newly qualified nurse, miscalculated the amount of insulin her patient needed. She injected the patient, 85-year-old Margaret Thomas of Pontypool in Wales, with ten times the required dose. By the time Evans had realised her mistake several hours later, Margaret Thomas had died (Stokes, 2009). Miscalculations can clearly lead to serious health complications or even death for patients, and yet they are preventable human errors. As a nurse, you will need good numeracy skills in many aspects of your job. From weighing patients to calculating how quickly a drug needs to be administered via an intravenous infusion, accuracy is vital and mistakes can have devastating consequences. Many nurses and student nurses struggle with numeracy, and recently there has been a great deal of research into the possible reasons for and consequences of this (Jukes and Gilchrist, 2006; Weeks et al., 2000). This chapter takes you through the basic mathematics skills you will need in order to carry out your day-to-day duties. It looks at the mathematical processes themselves, and at how to apply these to real situations involving medicines administration.

Using calculators and estimating answers

Although you may feel quite comfortable with using a calculator, it is vital that you understand the mathematics you are using and can work out answers without relying on one. There may not always be a calculator to hand, and although they may save you time and allow you to quickly check your answer, you need to understand what you are calculating rather than simply putting numbers into a machine. There will always be another nurse with whom you can check your answers; however, you should not be relying on *their* grasp of numeracy but on your own. Every nurse needs to be able to work medicine doses out by themselves, competently and reasonably quickly (NMC, 2007).

It is also worth mentioning estimation at this point, because you will inevitably need to use your judgement when calculating drug doses – does the answer you have come up with look reasonable? Most tablets, for example, are manufactured in a variety of strengths, and you may not find one that is exactly the strength you require. Maybe you will need to give the patient three of the tablets you have in stock. However, if you have calculated the dose and found that you need to give the patient thirty of these tablets, you will, hopefully, be able to use your judgement and think that this seems like a rather large pile of tablets to be giving the patient in one dose. If you come up with an answer that seems unlikely or unreasonable, it is probable that you have made a mistake somewhere in your calculations. You will need to check your working out to find where you went wrong. If you have used a calculator, it is impossible to tell where the mistake has been made – in fact, many people assume that the answer must be correct because the calculator has provided it. Calculators cannot tell whether you have entered the correct numbers in the correct order, so it is vital that you understand the process you are going through in order to reach your answer, and that you can judge whether that answer seems reasonable.

How to use this chapter

You may feel that your numeracy skills are already good, and that you only need to skim through this section of the book. You might be competent in some areas, but not in others. It may be many years since you studied mathematics at school; you may not have enjoyed it or you may have found it difficult. It is natural to feel nervous about using a skill you are not completely confident with, particularly when accuracy is so important to your patients' health. Whatever your starting point, you should be able to find useful information and activities in this chapter that will help you to prepare yourself for the kinds of calculations you will need to perform as a nurse.

Activity 1.1   *Reflection*

Assess your own numeracy skills: how confident do you feel with the following?

- adding and subtracting whole numbers;
- multiplication and division sums;
- understanding decimals: what they mean and adding, subtracting, multiplying and dividing decimals;
- converting between units, such as changing millilitres to litres and so on;
- ratios and strengths of solutions;
- working out how many tablets or how much liquid is required in order to fill a prescription;
- how a patient's weight might affect the dose you are required to administer for some medicines.

As this answer is based on your self-assessment, there is no outline answer at the end of the chapter.

As a nurse, you will need to be confident in all of the areas mentioned in the above activity. This chapter will look at each of them in turn.

What numbers are worth

Place value

The position of each **digit** within a larger number shows exactly what that digit is worth. You may remember using 'place value columns' at school, and these are useful tools when determining exactly what the value of each individual digit is. For example, if we take the number 482 and put it into a place value chart, it looks like this:

```
H   T   U
4   8   2
```

H stands for 'hundreds'	100
T stands for 'tens'	10
U stands 'units' (which means 'ones')	1

So, we can see that the number 482 is made up of four 'hundreds', eight 'tens' and two 'units'. The number 52,304 would fit into a place value chart like this:

```
TTh   Th   H   T   U
5     2    3   0   4
```

TTh stands for 'tens of thousands'	10,000
Th stands for 'thousands'	1000
H stands for 'hundreds'	100
T stands for 'tens'	10
U stands for 'units'	1

In this example, the number 52,304 is made up of five 'tens of thousands', two 'thousands', three 'hundreds', no tens and four 'units'. The zero in the 'tens' column is known as a place holder, and it is very important that we remember to include this zero – without it, many of the other digits would end up in the wrong columns and the number would represent a very different amount. Try the following activity to check how well you understand place value.

Activity 1.2

Work out the answers to the following questions:

1. Which number appears in the 'thousands' column of a place value chart for the number 562,103?
2. Write this number out in words: 24,086,079.
3. Write this number out in digits: three million, two hundred thousand, six hundred and fifty.
4. In the number 41,204,392, in which column of a place value chart would the digit 1 appear?
5. In the same number 41,204,392, in which column would the zero appear?

The answers to this activity can be found at the end of the chapter.

Decimals

Decimals or decimal fractions represent part of whole numbers. We experience decimals every day, when we use money. Four pounds and twelve pence would be written as £4.12. The whole numbers in this case are pounds. Everything after the decimal point represents a small part of a whole number and everything before the decimal point represents a whole number, so in this case there are four whole units before the decimal point (the four pounds). In the same way as before, the number can be fitted into a place value chart in order to show the true values of the digits that appear after the decimal point:

U	.	1/10	1/100
4	.	1	2

1/10 means one 'tenth', or one out of ten
1/100 means one 'hundredth', or one out of one hundred

In order to work out exactly what the 1 and 2 represent, we need to look at the column headings. In this case, there is one 'tenth' of a whole, and two 'hundredths'. Imagine something has been divided into ten equal parts – each one is called a tenth. Using money, this means that a pound has been divided into ten 10p pieces, and we have one of those pieces. Similarly, a pound can also be divided into one hundred hundredths (pence or pennies), and we have two of them. Imagining our £4.12 laid out in front of you using these coins, you would have four pound coins, one ten pence coin and two pennies. It can often help to imagine money when dealing with decimals, to help you to understand the quantities you are dealing with. Look at the next example:

H	T	U	.	1/10	1/100	1/1000
3	4	6	.	9	2	3

The number 346.923 is made up of the following:

- three hundreds;
- four tens;
- six units;
- nine tenths;
- two hundredths;
- three thousandths.

You would say it as 'three hundred and forty-six point nine two three'.

Just as with whole numbers, decimal numbers sometimes require a place holder zero to show that there is nothing in one of the columns. Again, without this zero, the number would mean something quite different as some of the digits would be in the wrong columns. For example:

T	U	.	1/10	1/100
2	0	.	0	4

This number is 20.04 or 'twenty point zero four'. It represents two tens, no units, no tenths and four hundredths. It may help to imagine this amount as money, £20.04. If you forgot to put the zero place holder in the units column, for example, the number would become £2.04, which is a very different amount to have in your pocket.

Activity 1.3

Answer the following questions:

1. Write 'fourteen pounds and three pence' out using digits in a place value chart.
2. What does the digit 6 represent in the number 128.46?
3. In which place value column does the digit 7 appear in the number 4.107?
4. Which of these numbers is bigger: 1.2 or 1.09?

The answers to this activity can be found at the end of the chapter.

Multiplying by 10, by 100 or by 1000

We know that $6 \times 10 = 60$. What is happening to the place value chart when we multiply 6 by 10?

```
T   U
    6
        ↓ × 10
6   0
```

The 6 has moved one place to the left into the tens column, and a place holder zero has been written in the units column as there are no units. Similarly, we know that $2 \times 100 = 200$, but how does this look in a place value chart?

```
H   T   U
        2
            ↓ × 100
2   0   0
```

This time, the 2 has moved two places to the left into the hundreds column, and the tens and units columns now both have place holder zeros in them. Do you notice the pattern? There is one zero in 10, so when multiplying by 10 we need to move one place to the left. There are two zeros in 100, so when multiplying by 100 we move our digits two places to the left. There are three zeros in 1000, so if we multiply our original number by 1000, it will move three places to the left, and so on.

Activity 1.4

Try the following questions:

1. 3×1000
2. 29×100
3. 86×10
4. $3,462 \times 100$
5. 70×1000

The answers to this activity can be found at the end of the chapter.

This works in exactly the same way when multiplying decimals. For example, 7.6×10 would look like this:

```
T   U   .   1/10
    7   .   6
                ↓ × 10
7   6   .   0
```

The answer is 76 (you do not need to write 76.0).
Similarly, 29.027×100 would be:

```
Th   H   T   U   .   1/10   1/100   1/1000
         2   9   .   0      2       7
                                      ↓ × 100
2    9   0   2   .   7
```

We have multiplied by 100, so everything has moved two columns to the left. The answer is 2902.7.

Dividing by 10, by 100 or by 1000

We know that $70 \div 10 = 7$. Demonstrating this using a place value chart shows us that all digits have now moved one place to the right:

```
T   U
7   0
        ↓ ÷ 10
    7
```

Dividing by 100 will mean that everything moves two places to the right, so $300 \div 100 = 3$ like this:

```
H   T   U
3   0   0
            ↓ ÷ 100
        3
```

This rule also works with decimals, for example $36 \div 10 = 3.6$ as shown below:

```
T   U   .   1/10
3   6   .   0
                ↓ ÷ 10
    3   .   6
```

Similarly, $12.04 \div 100 = 0.1204$ as shown below (all digits have moved two places to the right):

```
T   U   .   1/10   1/100   1/1000   1/10,000
1   2   .   0      4
                                    ↓ ÷ 100
    0   .   1      2       0        4
```

Activity 1.6

Try the following questions:

1. $24 \div 10$
2. $3.6 \div 100$
3. $62.64 \div 10$
4. $0.3 \div 100$
5. $12 \div 1000$

The answers to this activity can be found at the end of the chapter.

A quicker way of working

You may feel that you do not want or need to draw a place value chart every time you want to multiply or divide by 10, by 100 or by 1000. Many people find that, once they have grasped the concept, it is quicker and easier to concentrate on moving the decimal point rather than moving all of the digits within a chart. Using this quick method, you are imagining rather than drawing the place value columns. To demonstrate, here are the two methods of working out 0.6×10:

Using place value columns

```
U   .   1/10
0   .   6
            ↓ × 10
6   .   0
←_____
```

Digit moves one place to the left. The answer is 6.

Moving the decimal point

```
0.6     × 10
0 6.0
→
```

Decimal point moves one place to the right. The answer is 6.

If there is no decimal point in the original number, insert it where it should be (for example, 12 becomes 12.0). This allows you to move it as required. This example shows 12×100 using the quick method of moving the decimal point:

$$12.0 \times 100 \text{ becomes } 1200.0$$
$$\rightarrow$$

The decimal point has moved two places to the right and the answer is 1200. Remember to fill any empty place value columns with zeros so that the digits are in the correct columns.

Similarly, $4.07 \div 10$ can be worked out using this quick method:

$$0.407$$
$$\leftarrow$$

The decimal point has moved one place to the left, and we have filled in the units column with a place holder zero. You can check these calculations using place value columns if you prefer.

Activity 1.7

Answer the following questions using whichever method feels most comfortable:

1. $2.4 \div 100$
2. 6.092×10
3. $0.3 \div 1000$
4. 0.3×1000
5. $92.1 \div 100$
6. $16 \div 1000$
7. 1.5×100
8. $0.0032 \div 10$
9. 8.408×100
10. $24{,}609.37 \div 1000$

The answers to this activity can be found at the end of the chapter.

SI units

The UK's healthcare system uses the International System of Units, otherwise known as the *Système International d'Unités* or SI units. This system was introduced in Britain in 1975. SI units are used when measuring weights, lengths, quantities of liquids and so on, to ensure that a unified standard is in use around the world and that everyone understands which units to use. SI units are used in almost every country for scientific and healthcare purposes. In this chapter, we will look at the units and quantities that you are most likely to encounter as a nurse. You will need SI units for measuring length (such as a patient's height), weight (of patients or tablets) and volume of liquids.

Length

The standard unit for measuring length is the metre, which is usually shortened to m (for example, twelve metres would be written as 12m). There are numerous related units which you need to be aware of:

- one kilometre (1km)   =   one thousand metres (1000m)
- one metre (1m)   =   one hundred centimetres (100cm)
- one centimetre (1cm)   =   ten millimetres (10mm)
- one metre (1m)   =   one thousand millimetres (1000mm)

Weight

Weights are measured using the gram (g). Again, there are numerous related units:

- one kilogram (1kg)   =   one thousand grams (1000g)
- one gram (1g)   =   one thousand milligrams (1000mg)
- one milligram (1mg)   =   one thousand micrograms (1000mcg)

Note: micrograms are sometimes written as µg, but this looks very similar to mg which stands for milligrams (particularly when handwritten). Therefore, most people tend to write micrograms as mcg to avoid confusion, or you may even choose to write the word 'micrograms' out in full.

Liquids

Liquids are measured using the litre (shortened to l or L).

- one litre (1L)   =   one thousand millilitres (1000ml)

Converting between units

As a nurse, you will need to know how to convert between related units, such as from millilitres to litres or from milligrams to micrograms. This is because prescriptions may, for example, specify a dose in milligrams, but the box of capsules on the shelf may describe the contents in micrograms. You will therefore need to know whether the box contains the correct strength of tablets, and you will do this by converting between related units.

Scenario

You have been asked to find 2000ml of saline solution, and the stock is all in one-litre bags. How many do you need?

We know that one litre = 1000ml. So we can multiply each side of this equation by two to reach our desired quantity of 2000ml (we must multiply both sides of the equation so that they are both still equal to each other):

$$1 \text{ litre} = 1000\text{ml}$$
$$\downarrow \times 2 \qquad\qquad\qquad \downarrow \times 2$$
$$2 \text{ litres} = 2000\text{ml}$$

So to find 2000ml of the saline solution, you will need two of the one-litre bags.

However, it may not always be quite so straightforward. You might be asked to measure out 0.625 litres of the solution, but if your measuring scale is in millilitres, you will need to convert this amount from litres into millilitres in order to measure accurately. Again, we know that one litre = 1000ml. So to get from 1 to 1000 we have multiplied by 1000. To measure out 0.625L, we need to convert this into millilitres by multiplying by 1000.

$$0.625 \times 1000 = 625$$

To multiply by 100, the decimal point has been moved three places to the right. Therefore 0.625L = 625ml.

Activity 1.8

Using the information above and the techniques we looked at previously, work out the following conversions.

1. Convert 0.3 litres into millilitres.
2. Convert 36.7 litres into millilitres.
3. Convert 2.6L into ml.

The answers to this activity can be found at the end of the chapter.

Using the techniques shown earlier for multiplying and dividing by 10, by 100 and by 1000, you will be able to convert between any of the units mentioned. Table 1.1 sums up the calculations you will need.

The next activity tests how well you have grasped the topics we have looked at so far. You can use the table provided in Table 1.1 to help you if you need it. However, be aware that you may not have a chart like this handy in your day-to-day activities.

Activity 1.9

Answer the following questions:

1. Convert 25mm to cm.
2. Convert 3.2L to ml.
3. Convert 1.91m to cm.
4. Convert 86kg to g.
5. Convert 75mcg to mg.
6. Convert 0.2 mg to mcg.
7. You have 250ml of water. How many litres is this?
8. A patient is prescribed 30mg of codeine phosphate. How many grams is this?
9. You have a 500mg paracetamol tablet in front of you. How many mcg is this?
10. A patient requires 0.1mg of levothyroxine per day. How many micrograms is this?

The answers to this activity can be found at the end of the chapter.

Table 1.1: Calculations required when converting between SI units

Length

Converting from	Calculation	To
km	× 1000	m
m	÷ 1000	km
m	× 100	cm
cm	÷ 100	m
cm	× 10	mm
mm	÷ 10	cm
m	× 1000	mm
mm	÷ 1000	m

Weight

Converting from	Calculation	To
kg	× 1000	g
g	÷ 1000	kg
g	× 1000	mg
mg	÷ 1000	g
mg	× 1000	mcg
mcg	÷ 1000	mg

Volume of liquids

Converting from	Calculation	To
L	× 1000	ml
ml	÷ 1000	L

Addition

You will need to be able to add quantities together, including those that are given in different units, such as adding litres and millilitres. You might therefore need to convert between units before you can even begin adding, and it is vital that you check which units you are using before coming up with an answer, as dosage mistakes could have very serious consequences.

Adding whole numbers

When adding two or more numbers together, it is important to place each digit in the correct place value column, so that each number is worth the correct amount. You can then add the numbers in each column together, starting on the right with the units column and continuing column by column towards the left. For example, $32 + 16$ would be carried out like this:

```
    3   2
+   1   6
    4   8
        ↑
```

You have added $2 + 6$ in the units column (which equals 8) and then moved towards the left and added the $3 + 1$ in the tens column (which equals 4). The answer is therefore four tens and eight units, which is 48.

Sometimes, the answer you get in one column comes to more than ten, and you can only fit one digit in each column in your answer area. In the next example, you need to add 23 and 29 together. Adding the 3 and the 9 in the units column comes to 12. There are two digits in 12, so it cannot fit into the units column in your answer area. The 12 can be split into its constituent parts of 10 and 2. So, the 2 (units) is written in the units answer area, and the 1 (meaning 'one lot of ten') is 'carried over' into the tens column. It can then be added along with the other digits in the tens column, so that the answer contains the correct amount of tens.

```
    2   3
+   2   9
    5₁  2
        ↑
```

The small digit 1 in the tens column has been carried over from the units column ($2 + 2 = 4$, add the 1 brings us to 5). You may be used to writing this digit in a different place in your working out – this is fine, you may write it wherever you are used to writing it, as long as you remember to add it on.

Adding with decimals

You may need to add decimal fractions to each other or to whole numbers. Again, it is very important that each digit is written in the correct place value column. The addition itself works in exactly the same way as shown above, starting from the column on the right and moving towards the left. You may need to insert some zeros as place holders in order to line up your place value columns and avoid mistakes. For example, to work out the sum $2.4 + 30.17$:

These zeros have been added to make the sum easier to calculate.

```
    0   2   .   4   0
+   3   0   .   1   7
    3   2   .   5   7
```

As previously mentioned, you may need to convert between different units before you begin the sum itself, as you can only add quantities together that are given in the same unit. For example, a patient takes two paracetamol tablets, one weighing 0.5g and the other weighing 250mg. What is the total weight taken by the patient?

You cannot add 0.5g and 250mg together immediately, as grams and milligrams are very different in size. So you need to convert into the same units before you can begin adding. In this example, you have not been asked to give your answer in a particular unit, so it does not matter which units you choose to work with. Both answers are shown below.

By converting into grams
To convert 250mg into grams, we need to divide by 1000 (you can check this using the chart provided in Table 1.1).

$250 \div 1000 = 0.25$

We now need to add 0.25 to 0.5 (both numbers are now in grams).

```
    0  .  2  5
+   0  .  5  0
_____
    0  .  7  5
```

The answer is 0.75g.

By converting into milligrams
To convert 0.5g into mg, we need to multiply by 1000.

$0.5 \times 1000 = 500$

So 0.5g = 500mg

We now need to add 250mg and 500mg, which gives us 750mg.

The answer is therefore 750mg.

Both answers are the same, because 750mg = 0.75g. Be careful to give your answer in the correct units.

Activity 1.10

Work out the answers to the following:

1. $34.6 + 9.25$
2. You have 2.5 litres of water and add another 75ml to it. How much water do you now have? (Give your answer in litres.)
3. What is 2.5mg + 350mcg? (Give your answer in mcg.)

The answers to this activity can be found at the end of the chapter.

Subtraction

You may need to subtract one quantity from another – otherwise known as 'taking away'. As with addition, it is very important that each digit is written in the correct place value column. For example, $42 - 31$ would be written like this:

```
    4  2
-   3  1
_____
    1  1
```

Again, you need to start with the right-hand column and subtract the bottom digit from the top digit. In this example, you will therefore need to work out 2 − 1 first, then 4 − 3.

Sometimes, as in the next example of 732 − 514, you may not be able to carry out the subtraction immediately, as you cannot take 4 away from 2. In this case, you need to 'borrow' a ten from the tens column as shown, and take 4 away from 12 instead.

$$
\begin{array}{r}
7 \quad 3^2 \quad {}^{1}2 \\
-\ 5 \quad 1 \quad 4 \\
\hline
2 \quad 1 \quad 8
\end{array}
$$

In the example above, we have 'borrowed' a ten from the tens column (the 3 has therefore become a 2 as there are now two tens not three). We have then moved this ten into the units column, making it hold twelve rather than two.

Note: you may be more used to using a different method of subtraction, and it is important that you use the method with which you feel most comfortable. The most common alternative method is called 'paying back', whereby the ten is not removed from the top row of the tens column but is 'paid back' to the bottom row instead. The answer will be exactly the same, and the above sum would look like this:

$$
\begin{array}{r}
7 \quad 3 \quad {}^{1}2 \\
-\ 5 \quad {}^{2}1 \quad 4 \\
\hline
2 \quad 1 \quad 8
\end{array}
$$

Subtraction with decimals

As with addition, you subtract decimals in exactly the same way as you would subtract whole numbers. Make sure that your place value columns are lined up correctly, which may mean that you need to insert place holder zeros such as in the next example.

Work out the answer to 34− 22.8. You would set the sum out like this:

$$
\begin{array}{r}
3 \quad 4^3 \quad . \quad {}^{1}0 \\
-\ 2 \quad 2 \quad . \quad 8 \\
\hline
1 \quad 1 \quad . \quad 2
\end{array}
$$

The answer is therefore 11.2.

Remember that you may need to convert between units before subtracting.

Activity 1.11

Try the following questions, using whichever method you find most comfortable.

1. 53.9 − 14.21
2. You have three litres of water and you use 25ml of it. How much is left, in millilitres?
3. At their first appointment, a patient weighs 82.5kg. By their second appointment, they weigh 76.25kg. How many grams have they lost?

The answers to this activity can be found at the end of the chapter.

Multiplication

Multiplication skills are essential when calculating drug doses. You will probably find it useful to practise your times tables (up to ten) before attempting this section, as long multiplication depends on them. You may be able to say your times tables in your head or out loud, or you might prefer to write them down. You might even feel more comfortable carrying a multiplication square around with you, like the one in Table 1.2, if you find your tables hard to remember. If you are struggling with them, think about what multiplication means and how you could fill in any gaps. For example, if you can remember that $6 \times 6 = 36$, but cannot recall 7×6, you can work out the answer by adding on another 6 to 36. Multiplication can be thought of as repeated addition: 3×2 can be thought of as 'three twos' or 'three lots of two'. As it involves small numbers, it can easily be worked out by repeatedly adding:

$$
\begin{array}{r}
2 \\
+ \quad 2 \\
2 \\
\hline
6
\end{array}
$$

Therefore, $3 \times 2 = 6$.

You can use this technique for helping you with your times tables or for working out smaller sums such as this one.

You have two tablets, each weighing 25mg. What is the total weight of the tablets? To answer this by repeated addition is easy:

$$
\begin{array}{r}
2 \quad 5 \\
+ \quad 2 \quad 5 \\
\hline
5 \quad 0
\end{array}
$$

The answer is 50g.

However, this method would be very difficult and time-consuming for larger quantities. Imagine you have 65 of those 25mg tablets – to answer this using repeated addition would take an incredibly long time and there would be a much greater chance of making a mistake. Using other multiplication techniques makes such calculations far easier and less time-consuming.

Multiplying larger numbers by single-digit whole numbers

You have some tablets weighing 125mcg each. You weigh out nine of them – what will the total weight be?

This can be worked out by multiplying 125 by 9, and you would write it out like this:

$$
\begin{array}{r}
1 \quad 2 \quad 5 \\
\times \quad \quad 9 \\
\hline
\end{array}
$$

The 125 is made up of 5, 20 and 100, or five units, two tens and one hundred.

Table 1.2: Multiplication square

×	1	2	3	4	5	6	7	8	9	10
1	1	2	3	4	5	6	7	8	9	10
2	2	4	6	8	10	12	14	16	18	20
3	3	6	9	12	15	18	21	24	27	30
4	4	8	12	16	20	24	28	32	36	40
5	5	10	15	20	25	30	35	40	45	50
6	6	12	18	24	30	36	42	48	54	60
7	7	14	21	28	35	42	49	56	63	70
8	8	16	24	32	40	48	56	64	72	80
9	9	18	27	36	45	54	63	72	81	90
10	10	20	30	40	50	60	70	80	90	100

Starting with the units column, you then multiply each column in turn by nine. So, you work out 5×9, then 2×9, and then 1×9.

$$
\begin{array}{r}
1 \quad 2 \quad 5 \\
\times \qquad\quad 9 \\
\hline
1 \quad 1_2 \ 2_4 \ 5
\end{array}
$$

You will have gone through these stages:

- Work out 5×9. The answer is 45. As before, only one digit can fit in each column of the answer area, so the 5 is written in the answer area and the 4 (representing four tens or forty) is carried into the tens column to be added onto the answer there.
- Work out 2×9. The answer is 18. You then need to add the 4 you carried over, making a total of 22. Your answer for this column is 22 – as before, you need to carry the 2, which represents 20, into the next column, where it will be added to the answer for that column.
- Work out $1 \times 9 = 9$. You need to add the 2 you carried over, making a total of 11. As there are no more columns to multiply, you write 11 in the thousands and hundreds columns of the answer area.
- Your answer is 1125mcg. You have one thousand, one hundred (or eleven hundreds), one twenty and five units.
- Always remember which units you are using.

Multiplying decimals by single-digit whole numbers

In this example, you have nine tablets, each weighing 1.55mg. What is the total weight of all nine tablets?

Multiplying with decimals is the one area where it is advisable *not* to write the sum out in strict place value columns. Instead, you will probably find it easier to ignore the decimal point at first (we will come back to it later). So, to work out this sum, you would need to do this:

$$
\begin{array}{r}
1 \ \ .5 \ \ 5 \\
\times \qquad \quad 9 \\
\hline
1 \ \ 3_4 \ \ .9_4 \ \ 5 \ \ \text{mg}
\end{array}
$$

You will go through these stages:

- Work out the sum as if the decimal point was not there at first.
- $5 \times 9 = 45$ (carry the 4 into the next column).
- $5 \times 9 = 45$, then add on the 4 you carried over, which gives you 49. Carry the 4 into the next column.
- $1 \times 9 = 9$, then add the 4 you carried over, $9 + 4 = 13$.
- You now have 1395. You need to replace the decimal point in the correct position. The trick to doing so is this: work out how many digits there are in the sum *after* the decimal point. In this example there are two (the two fives). You need the same number of digits after the decimal point in your answer, so replace the decimal point two places in from the right in your answer. In this case, this gives you 13.95.
- Your final answer is therefore 13.95mg.

This trick also includes any zeros in your answer, such as in the sum below – there are two digits after the decimals point in the question (3 and 4) so you need to have two digits after the decimal point in your answer (the 7 and 0 will be after the decimal point).

$$
\begin{array}{r}
2 \ \ .3 \ \ 4 \\
\times \qquad \quad 5 \\
\hline
1 \ \ 1_1 \ \ .7_2 \ \ 0
\end{array}
$$

Try the questions in the activity below before moving on to the next section. Be careful to give your answer in the correct units.

Activity 1.12

Answer the following questions, using multiplication:

1. A patient is prescribed 250mg of carisoprodol, four times a day for three days. How much carisoprodol will the patient take in total, in grams?
2. A patient takes two 0.075g tablets of amoxicillin. How many milligrams do they take in total?

The answers to this activity can be found at the end of the chapter.

Long multiplication

Long multiplication is used when multiplying numbers of more than one digit by other numbers of more than one digit. There are several methods of doing this, and the most common is described here. If you are comfortable using a different method, you can continue using it when trying the activities in this section. For example, we will work out the answer to 73×24:

```
    7   3
×   2   4
_____
```

You cannot work this out immediately as the numbers are too big, so you need to break 24 into its constituent parts of 20 and 4. You can then multiply, in effect, 73 by 20 and then by 4. Adding these two answers together will give you the final answer to the original sum. It makes no difference in which order you do this (multiplying by the 20 first or by the 4), but as you may be used to working in only one of these ways, both are shown here.

Multiplying by the 4 first

```
            7    3
        ×   2    4
        _____
        2   9₁   2
+   1   4   6    0
    _____
    1   7₁  5    2
```

You must insert this zero to show that you are multiplying by 20, not by 2. This zero moves all of the digits into their correct place value columns.

You will have gone through the following stages:

- $3 \times 4 = 12$ (carry the 1 into the next column).
- $7 \times 4 = 28$. Add the 1 you carried over, making 29.
- Move on to multiplying by 20 – insert a zero to show that you are actually multiplying by 20, not by 2. You then continue to multiply each column by 2.
- $3 \times 2 = 6$.
- $7 \times 2 = 14$.
- You now have two answers. You know that $73 \times 4 = 292$, and $73 \times 20 = 1460$. You need to add them together to find the total, which will give you the answer to 73×24.
- $292 + 1460 = 1752$. Your answer is 1752.

Multiplying by the 20 first

```
                7    3
            ×   2    4
            _____
        1   4   6    0
+           2   9₁   2
    _____
    1   7₁  5    2
```

As you can see, this gives exactly the same answer, as you have carried out the same calculation but in a very slightly different order. In this case, you have multiplied by the 20 first, so you need to put your zero place holder in the first answer row to show that you are multiplying by 20. As before, you then multiply 3×2, followed by 7×2. In the next stage, you multiply by the 4 (3×4, then 7×4). Again, adding the two answers you have come up with will give you the final answer ($1460 + 292 = 1752$).

Long multiplication with decimals

As shown before, it is often best to ignore the decimal point at first when multiplying with decimals. When you have reached an answer, replace the decimal point in the correct location to make sure that all digits are in the correct place value columns. For example, we need to find the answer to 28×1.5. Work out 28×15 first, then look to see how many digits appear after the decimal point in the original sum (in this sum, one digit appears after the decimal point). Place your decimal point so that the same number of digits appear after it (in this case, one).

$$
\begin{array}{r r r}
 & 2 & 8 \\
\times & 1 & .5 \\
\hline
2 & 8 & 0 \\
+ \quad 1 & 4_4 & 0 \\
\hline
4_1 & 2 & .0 \\
\end{array}
$$

The answer is 42.0, which can then be shortened to 42. You can estimate whether your answer looks plausible – you are looking for one-and-a-half times twenty-eight, so you know that the answer is not going to be 420 or 4.2 (decimal point replaced in wrong place).

Worked example

Find the answer to 9.34×6.1.

$$
\begin{array}{r r r r r}
 & 9 & .3 & 4 \\
 & \times & 6 & .1 \\
\hline
5 & 6_2 & 0_2 & 4 & 0 \\
+ \quad & & 9 & 3 & 4 \\
\hline
5 & 6 & .9 & 7 & 4 \\
\end{array}
$$

In this sum, there are three digits after the decimal point (the three, the four and the one) so there must be three digits after the decimal point in the answer too. The answer is 56.974.

The questions in the activity below will give you the opportunity to practise using long multiplication. You can use a calculator to check your answers, but you need to be able to carry out these kinds of calculations without one.

Activity 1.13

Answer the following, using whichever method of long multiplication you like:

1. 126×38
2. 96×2.3
3. 3.82×4.1
4. A patient takes one bisoprolol 3.75mg tablet each day. How many milligrams will they take in a week?

5. Your patient is prescribed 1.75mg of lorazepam, three times a day. How much (in grams) will the patient take in a five-day period?

The answers to this activity can be found at the end of the chapter.

As mentioned earlier, you should use your judgement as to whether an answer looks right. You can get a rough idea of what the answer will be by estimating or rounding numbers. For example, if you need to work out 2.1 × 3.9, you could round it to 2 × 4 (2.1 is almost 2 and 3.9 is almost 4). You know that the answer therefore needs to be somewhere close to 8, and the correct answer is in fact 8.19. You can judge that your answer of 8.19 is likely to be correct as it is about right, whereas if you had come up with an answer of 81.9 you would be able to see that you had made a mistake.

Division

Division is often called 'sharing' as it is easiest to explain in terms of sharing one quantity with another. For example, you have a pizza that is cut into eight equal slices. You share it equally between four people – how many slices does each person receive? This one is easy, as you can visualise eight slices divided by four people. 8 ÷ 4 = 2. You can check your answer by multiplying the two slices each by the four people, that is 2 × 4 = 8. However, larger sums may be more difficult, and this is where various methods of short and long division will be useful. There are many different ways of dividing, and the most common is shown here (again, if you are comfortable with another method, you may use it to calculate the answers to the questions in this section).

Worked example

A patient is prescribed 75mg per day of their medicine. This needs to be spread between three equal doses at meal times. How large is each single dose?

To answer this question, you need to divide 75 by 3. You could write this out as 75 ÷ 3, but you may not be able to work it out in that way. You are probably familiar with division sums that look like this:

$$3 \overline{)7 \quad 5}$$

This means 75 divided by 3, or how many threes there are in seventy-five. Working out this sum step by step gives us an answer of 25mg.

$$3 \overline{)7 \quad {}^{1}5} \quad \begin{array}{cc} 2 & 5 \end{array}$$

You will need to carry out these stages:

*   Starting with the column on the left this time, you need to find out how many threes there are in seven.

Worked example continued

- The answer is two, so the digit 2 is placed above the 7 in the answer area. However, $3 \times 2 = 6$, so there is one left over. This needs to be 'carried over' into the next column, so the five becomes fifteen (you have actually been finding out how many threes there are in seventy, as the seven is in the tens column, so there is one ten left over. That is why the five becomes fifteen – you have carried a ten into the units column).
- Now you need to find out how many threes there are in fifteen – there are five, so the digit 5 is written in the answer area.
- Your answer to the sum is 25, as $75 \div 3 = 25$.
- Remember you are working in milligrams, so each dose will weigh 25mg.

Dividing by two-digit numbers

This works in exactly the same way, even though it looks more complicated. For example, to find the answer to $144 \div 12$, you can do the following:

$$\begin{array}{r} 0\ \ 1\ \ 2 \\ 12\overline{)\ 1\ \ 4\ \ {}^{2}4} \end{array}$$

- How many twelves are there in one? This cannot be done, so we place a zero in the answer area and carry the one over into the next column.
- We now need to know how many twelves there are in fourteen. There is one, so we place a digit 1 in the answer area. There are also two left over, which we carry across into the next column.
- How many twelves are there in twenty-four? There are exactly two, so we place a digit 2 in our answer area, giving us a final answer of 12.
- Therefore, $144 \div 12 = 12$.

Remainders

Sometimes, the answer might not be as straightforward as in the examples above. One number might not divide exactly into the other, and you may have a quantity 'left over' – a remainder. As a nurse, you will always need to work out your answer accurately and give your answers as decimals, rather than something like 'four remainder one'. Bear in mind that 'four remainder one' is unlikely to equate to 4.1, so you will need to be able to work out answers to these kinds of questions accurately. The example below shows how you can work out the answer to $68 \div 8$.

$$\begin{array}{r} 0\ \ 8\ \ .\ \ 5 \\ 8\overline{)\ 6\ \ 8\ \ .\ \ {}^{4}0} \end{array}$$

You need to go through these stages:

- How many eights in six? You cannot do this, so place a zero in the answer area.
- How many eights in sixty-eight? $8 \times 8 = 64$, so there are eight with four left over. Place the eight in the answer area and carry the four over to the next column.
- As there is no 'next column' yet, you need to insert the decimal point where it would be (68.0) and carry the four over so that the next column becomes 40. You are now looking for how many eights there are in forty.

- There are five eights in forty, with nothing left over. Remember to place the decimal point in the answer area, directly above the decimal point in the sum itself. Your answer is 8.5 (note that eight remainder four did not equate to eight point four).

Dividing whole numbers into decimal numbers

This works in exactly the same way as the example above. Imagine you need to divide 12.5mg of a medicine into four equal doses. You could work out the sum like this:

$$
\begin{array}{c}
0\quad 3\ .\ 1\quad 2\quad 5 \\
\hline
4\,|\,1\quad 2\ .\ 5\quad {}^{1}0\quad {}^{4}0
\end{array}
$$

- How many fours are there in twelve? There are three.
- How many fours are there in five? There is one, with one left over. You therefore need to carry the one into the next column and add another zero to the sum (12.5 becomes 12.50).
- You can then find out how many fours there are in ten. There are two, with two left over, so repeat the process of adding another zero.
- You are now looking for the number of fours in twenty. There are exactly five.
- Your answer is 3.125mg per dose.

The next activity gives you the opportunity to practise the kinds of division questions we have looked at so far.

Activity 1.14

Answer the following:

1. $186 \div 6$
2. $169 \div 13$
3. $103.5 \div 6$
4. $99.2 \div 8$
5. $21.35 \div 7$

The answers and working for this activity can be found at the end of the chapter.

Dividing by a decimal

We have already looked at dividing *into* a decimal number. However, you may need to divide *by* a decimal number. If you have a pile of tablets with a total weight of 15g, and you know that each tablet weights 2.5g, how can you use written division to find out how many tablets are in the pile? You need to calculate $15 \div 2.5$.

$$
2.5\,|\,1\quad 5
$$

However, finding out how many two-point-fives there are in another number is quite tricky. Ideally, we want to be dividing by a whole number, so we want to get rid of the decimal point. We cannot just remove it, but we can multiply each side of the sum by ten in order to get rid of the decimal point without changing the proportion of the sum. For example, $4 \div 2$ and $40 \div 20$ will give you exactly the same answer (two) – each 'side' of the sum has been multiplied by ten so the proportion of the sum remains the same. If we had only multiplied one side of the sum by ten but not the other, we would have ended up with either 40 ÷ 2 (which equals 20) or 2 ÷ 40 (which equals 0.05). These are both rather different answers. It is therefore vital that we multiply both sides of the sum when 'getting rid of' a decimal point in this way.

Therefore, our original sum of 15 ÷ 2.5 now becomes 150 ÷ 25. In this example, there are six tablets in the pile.

$$
\begin{array}{r}
0\ \ 0\ \ 6 \\
25\,\overline{)1\ \ 5\ \ 0}
\end{array}
$$

Activity 1.15

Answer the following questions using written methods of division:

1. 75 ÷ 1.2
2. A pack of tablets weighs 90mg, excluding the packaging. Each individual tablet weighs 1.5mg. How many tablets are in the pack?
3. A box containing capsules weighs 250g in its entirety. The box itself weighs 30g, and each capsule weighs 0.5g. How many capsules are in the box?

The answers to this activity can be found at the end of the chapter.

In the chapter so far, we have looked at addition, subtraction, multiplication and division (the 'four rules of number'). We have also looked at decimals and how to calculate with them, and at units of measure along with how to convert between them. There are a few more topics that you will need to be familiar with, and these are discussed below.

Ratios

Simply put, a **ratio** is the relationship between two quantities. Imagine you are making some orange squash. You use a cordial-to-water ratio of 1:4 (one to four). This means that for every one cup of cordial you use, you will need four cups of water. Similarly, for every 100ml of cordial used, there will be 400ml of water. If you use 250ml of cordial, you will need 1000ml (or one litre) of water, and the entire drink will measure 1.25 litres (1250ml).

Worked example

At a party, the ratio of men to women is 3:2. If there are 24 men at the party, how many women are there?

$$
\begin{array}{ccc}
\text{Men} & : & \text{Women} \\
3 & : & 2 \\
\times 8\downarrow & & \downarrow \times 8 \\
24 & : & 16
\end{array}
$$

We have multiplied the three by eight to get 24, so we must therefore multiply the two by eight as well – this gives us an answer of 16 women (and a total number of guests of 24 + 16 = 40).

You may come across ratios when diluting medicines or finding the correct strength drug. Many drugs are available in solutions of different strengths, and it is very important that you choose the correct one. Imagine the orange squash again. A cordial-to-water ratio of 1:4 means that there are five 'parts' to the mixture (one cup of cordial plus four cups of water equals five cups of liquid in total). Therefore, the cordial represents one out of the five parts, or 1/5, and may be referred to as a '1 in 5' solution (the cordial is one of the five parts). If we made our squash in a 1:10 ratio, it would be much weaker or less concentrated, as there would be eleven 'parts' and the cordial only represents one of them. This would be 1/11 or a one in eleven solution.

The same applies to medicines you will encounter as a nurse. A solution with a concentrate to water ratio of 1:100 is much stronger than a solution whose concentrate to water ratio is 1:10,000. As ever, you must be very careful with your units to ensure that you are finding the correct dose and have not confused your litres and millilitres.

You will probably see strengths of solutions written in the format mg/ml, or milligrams per millilitre. This refers to the amount of milligrams of active ingredient (drug) found in one millilitre of the solution. A solution with a strength of 5mg/ml has 5mg of the active ingredient in every millilitre of liquid. Therefore, ten millilitres of the solution will provide fifty milligrams of the drug itself. We will return to calculations using quantities like this shortly.

Percentages

'Per cent' means 'out of one hundred', and refers to how much of something you have. For example, fifty-five **per cent** (55%) means fifty-five out of every hundred. It could also be written as a **fraction** (55/100), or as a decimal (0.55, meaning we have fifty-five hundredths). To find 55 per cent of something, you can multiply it by 0.55. To find 43 per cent, multiply by 0.43 and so on. You change the percentage into a decimal (how many hundredths do you have?) and multiply your original number by this decimal. For example, to find 25 per cent of 40, change the 25 per cent into a decimal (0.25) and multiply the original number by this. $0.25 \times 40 = 10$, so 25 per cent of 40 is 10.

As with ratios, you will probably see percentages used to describe the strengths of solutions. Looking at the orange squash example again, if the drink is made up of cordial and water, and cordial represents 10 per cent of the squash, water must make up 90 per cent (10% + 90% = 100%). Similarly, if dithranol ointment has a strength of 2 per cent, it means that 2g out of every 100g is the active ingredient. A 200g tube of ointment will contain 4g of active ingredient, and so on.

Drug strengths or concentrations may be expressed as:

- w/v (weight in volume) used when solids are dissolved in water to make solutions;
- w/w (weight in weight) when solids are dissolved in other solids, such as creams or ointments);
- v/v (volume in volume) when liquids are mixed into other liquids.

It is important to remember the following when calculating drug concentrations:

- one litre of water weighs one kilogram;
- one millilitre of water weighs one gram.

These weights are taken to be accurate for drug calculation purposes. So, a 20 per cent w/v solution means that 20g of a drug has been dissolved in every 100ml of water (20% = 20 out of 100, so if there is 20g of a drug dissolved, it must be in 100ml of water as 1g = 1ml).

Try the following questions, which are about ratio and percentages.

1. What weight, in grams, of glucose is dissolved in two litres of a solution with a strength of 10 per cent w/v?
2. How many grams of active ingredient are dissolved in 15ml of 5 per cent w/v solution?
3. How many grams of hydrocortisone are there in 200g of a cream with a strength of 1 per cent w/w?
4. Another batch of hydrocortisone cream is mixed with base ingredients to a ratio of 1:49. You have 100g of the cream. How many grams are of the active ingredient?
5. Which cream is stronger (contains more active ingredient): the cream in question 3 or the cream in question 4?

The answers to this activity can be found at the end of the chapter.

If you have found any of the questions so far difficult, it may help to read over again the relevant sections of this chapter before moving on.

Drug calculation formulae

You have already carried out many of the common calculations you will need as a nurse. There are some formulae with which you need to familiarise yourself, as they will be very useful to you in your career. However, as explained at the very beginning of this chapter, you cannot rely on trying to follow a formula simply by using a calculator. You need to understand the stages you are going through, and must be able to spot and correct any mistakes you make. This chapter so far has looked at the numeracy skills you will need and how to apply these to real situations. This section looks at the formulae that will help you, and how to use them effectively using the skills you have been developing.

How many tablets?

The formula for working out how many tablets or capsules you will need is as follows:

$$\frac{\text{Amount prescribed}}{\text{Amount available in each tablet}} = \text{number of tablets you need}$$

Worked example

A patient is prescribed 45mg of lansoprazole per day, to be taken in one dose. The available capsules contain 15mg each. How many capsules does the patient need to take?

$$\frac{45}{15} = 3$$

(45/15 means the same as 45 ÷ 15, or how many fifteens there are in forty-five.)
You can check this by working out 3 × 15 = 45.

How many tablets by body weight?

Sometimes you will need to calculate dosage according to the body weight of the patient. This is more common in children's nursing. This will be given in, say, milligrams per kilogram of body weight (mg/kg). The formula to help you is:

Body weight (kg) × dose per kg = dose required

Worked example

A patient is prescribed a dose of 10mg/kg, and they weigh 80kg. How much does the patient require?

$$80 \times 10 = 800mg$$

How much liquid?

The formula for calculating how much of a liquid you need is:

$$\frac{\text{Amount prescribed}}{\text{Amount available (strength)}} \times \text{volume the drug is in} = \text{required volume}$$

In other words:

$$\frac{\text{How much you need}}{\text{What strength you have}} \times \text{volume it's in} = \text{volume to give to patient}$$

You may be able to think of a simple way of remembering this formula, such as 'DRUG' (courtesy of Dawn L Hennefer):

$$\frac{\text{Dose Required}}{\text{what you've Got}} \times \text{Unit}$$

Worked example

You need to get a dose of aminophylline ready for a patient. Aminophylline is available in 250mg in 10ml (250mg of the active ingredient has been dissolved into every 10ml of the liquid), and you need 100mg of it. What volume of the solution is needed?

Worked example continued

$$\frac{100}{250} \times 10 =$$

Dividing first:

$$250 \overline{\smash{\big)}\ 1\ \ 0\ \ 0\ .\ 0} 0\ \ 0\ \ 0\ .\ 4$$

$$0.4 \times 10 = 4ml$$

Multiplying first:

$$100 \times 10 = 1000$$

$$1000 \div 250$$

$$= 250 \overline{\smash{\big)}\ 1\ \ 0\ \ 0\ \ 0} 0\ \ 0\ \ 0\ \ 4$$

$$= 4\ ml$$

There are two ways to continue from this point. You can either divide first, or multiply first. As you can see from the example given, for this formula it does not matter which part of the sum you do first – the answer is the same. You can therefore either multiply or divide first, depending on which you find easiest or on which numbers you have in your equation. We can demonstrate that this is the case for this formula by using simple numbers:

$$\frac{4}{2} \times 3 =$$

Dividing first:

$$4 \div 2 = 2$$

$$2 \times 3 = 6$$

Multiplying first:

$$4 \times 3 = 12$$

$$12 \div 2 = 6$$

How many drops per minute (for intravenous fluids)?

You may need to calculate the 'rate of flow' for medicines that are delivered directly into the bloodstream (see Chapter 4 for more information about these drugs). There are three common types of equipment that deliver **intravenous** fluids:

- the standard delivery or administration set, which delivers 20 drops per millilitre;
- the micro-drop delivery or administration set, which delivers 60 drops per millilitre;
- administration sets for giving blood, which give 15 drops per millilitre.

Be aware that you may also need to calculate rates for other equipment.
The formula to calculate the number of drops per minute (**dpm**) is:

$$\frac{\text{Millilitres to be given} \times \text{drops per ml}}{\text{Number of hours} \times 60} = \text{dpm}$$

The number of hours is multiplied by sixty as there are sixty minutes in an hour. The number of drops per millilitre is dependent on which administration equipment you are using. It is important that you do not confuse drops per millilitre and drops per minute (dpm).

Worked example

A patient is prescribed 400ml of glucose 5 per cent solution over two hours. You are using a standard administration set. Calculate the number of drops per minute. The example below shows how to work this out. The answer is 66.666 recurring, so we can round this up to 67 drops per minute. Notice that the strength of the solution (5 per cent) is irrelevant to our calculation.

$$\frac{400 \times 20}{2 \times 60} = \frac{800}{120} = 800 \div 120$$

$$(120 \times 6 = 720)$$

$$\begin{array}{r} 0\ \ 0\ \ 6\ \ \ \ 6\ .\ \ \ \ 6 \\ \hline 120\,\lvert\,8\ \ 0\ \ 0\ \ \ ^{80}0\ .\ \ ^{80}0 \end{array}$$

Activity 1.17

The following questions are designed to test your ability to answer realistic problems that you may face in your job, using the techniques, skills and formulae discussed throughout this chapter.

1. Digoxin tablets each weigh 62.5mcg. Your patient requires 0.25mg. How many tablets will you give the patient?
2. A patient requires 1.2g of penicillin intravenously. You have vials of penicillin available which each contain 600mg and require 2ml of water to be added to them in order to reconstitute the drug ready for injection. How many ml of water will you need for the entire dose?
3. Your patient needs 14mg of metoclopramide. The solution you have available contains 10mg in 2ml. How many ml will you need to give the patient, so that they receive the correct amount of the drug?
4. A patient is prescribed a hydrocortisone injection. The required dose is 20mg. The stock you have contains 50mg in 2ml. How much do you need to administer?
5. You need to prepare 0.25g of sulphasalazine. The available medicine is 500mg in 5ml. How much do you give the patient?
6. Your patient is prescribed tobramycin at 2mg/kg every eight hours. The patient weighs 85kg. How much in mg will they receive in a twenty-four hour period?
7. Morphine sulphate is prescribed as a dose of 20mg every 6 hours. Your ampoules contain 10mg in one ml. How much (in ml) will be given in twenty-four hours?
8. A patient takes 0.15mg of levothyroxine per day. You have 50mcg tablets available. How many tablets per day would you need to give the patient?
9. Using a standard administration set, how many drops per minute will be delivered for 0.3L of saline solution over three hours?
10. Using a micro-drop administration set, how many dpm will there be if 500ml of glucose 5 per cent is delivered over two-and-a-half hours?

The answers to this activity can be found at the end of the chapter.

In this chapter, we have looked at the numeracy skills you will need as a nurse, and at the kinds of calculations you will need to be able to do. We looked at place value, and how the position of each digit is vital in determining the value of a number. Using this knowledge, we then discussed how to multiply and divide by 10, by 100 and by 1000, before applying this to converting between SI units of measure. You have practised addition, subtraction, multiplication and division, with whole numbers and decimals. There was also information about ratio and percentages, and how these might be relevant to nursing. Finally, we studied the drug calculation formulae that will help you as a nurse, and used all of the techniques covered within the chapter to answer realistic questions using these formulae.

Activities: brief outline answers

Activity 1.2 (page 7)

1. 2
2. Twenty-four million, eighty-six thousand and seventy-nine. Written out with place value columns, this would be:

TM	M	HTh	TTh	Th	H	T	U
2	4	0	8	6	0	7	9

TM means 'tens of millions'
M means 'millions'
HTh means 'hundreds of thousands' and so on.
3. 3,200,650
4. The millions column (1,000,000).
5. The tens of thousands column (10,000).

Activity 1.3 (page 9)

1.
T	U	.	1/10	1/100
£1	4	.	0	3

2. It is in the 'hundredths' column, and represents six hundredths.
3. The thousandths column.
4. 1.2 is bigger, as it represents one whole number and two tenths. 1.09 represents one whole number and nine hundredths (hundredths are smaller than tenths). It may help you to visualise this if you think of the amounts as money, i.e. £1.20 and £1.09.

Activity 1.4 (page 9)

1. 3000
2. 2900
3. 860
4. 346,200
5. 70,000

Activity 1.5 (page 10)
1. 1250
2. 3490.4
3. 66,200

Activity 1.6 (page 11)
1. 2.4
2. 0.036
3. 6.264
4. 0.003
5. 0.012

Activity 1.7 (page 12)
1. 0.024
2. 60.92
3. 0.0003
4. 300
5. 0.921
6. 0.016
7. 150
8. 0.00032
9. 840.8
10. 24.60937

Activity 1.8 (page 14)
1. 300ml
2. 36,700ml
3. 2600ml

Activity 1.9 (page 14)
1. 2.5cm
2. 3200ml
3. 191cm
4. 86,000g
5. 0.075mg
6. 200mcg
7. 0.25L
8. 0.03g
9. 500,000mcg
10. 100mcg

Activity 1.10 (page 17)
1. 43.85
2. 75ml = 0.075L

```
   2 .  5
+  0 .  0  7  5
   2 .  5  7  5
```

The answer is 2.575 litres

3. 2.5mg = 2500mcg

```
  2   5   0   0
+ 3   5   0
─────────────
  2   8   5   0
```

The answer is 2850mcg

Activity 1.11 (page 18)

1.
```
  ⁴5  ¹3  .  ⁸9  ¹0
−  1   4  .   2   1
─────────────────
   3   9  .   6   9
```

The answer is 39.69.

2. 3 litres = 3000ml
   3000 − 25 = 2975

   The answer is 2975ml.

3. 82.50 − 76.25 = 06.25
   6.25kg = 6250g

   The answer is 6250g.

Activity 1.12 (page 21)

1. 250mg × 4 times a day = 1000mg
   1000mg × 3 days = 3000mg
   3000mg = 3g total dose

   The answer is 3g.

2. You can work this out in two ways:
   a) By converting g to mg first
      0.075g = 75mg
      75 × 2 = 150
      Total = 150mg
   b) By multiplying first
      0.075 × 2 = 0.150
      This is 0.15g.
      Convert to mg:
      0.15g = 150mg

Activity 1.13 (page 23)

1. 4788
2. 220.8
3. 15.662
4. 26.25mg
5. 0.02625g

Activity 1.14 (page 26)

1. 31
2. 13
3. 17.25
4. 12.4
5. 3.05
   The working out is shown here.

   (a)

   ```
         0  3  1
   6 | 1  8  6
   ```

   (b)

   ```
         0  1   3
   13 | 1  6  ³9
   ```

   (c)

   ```
         0  1  7  .  2   5
   6 | 1  0  ⁴3  .  ¹5  ³0
   ```

   (d)

   ```
        1   2  .   4
   8 | 9  ¹9  .  ³2
   ```

   (e)

   ```
        0  3  .  0  5
   7 | 2  1  .  3  5
   ```

Activity 1.15 (page 27)

1. 62.5
2. 60 tablets
3. 440 capsules
   The working out is shown here.

   (a)

   ```
   1.2 | 7   5
   ```

   ```
         0  6  2  .   5
   12 | 7  5  ³0  .  ⁶0
   ```

   (b)

   ```
   1.5 | 9   0
   ```

   ```
         0  6  0
   15 | 9  0  0
   ```

   (c)

250g	–	30g	=	220g
(total weight	–	weight of box	=	weight of capsules)

   ```
   0.5 | 2   2   0
   ```

$$
\begin{array}{r}
0\ \ 5\ \ 5\ \ 0 \\
5\overline{\smash{\big)}\ 2\ \ 2\ \ {}^{2}0\ \ 0}
\end{array}
$$

Activity 1.16 (page 29)

1. 2 litres = 2000ml. Divide by 10 to find 10% = 200ml. We know that 1ml = 1g, so there are 200g of glucose. The answer is 200g.
2. 15ml = 15g. We need 5 per cent of this. We know that 5% = 5/100 or five hundredths (0.05), so if we multiply 15 by 0.05 we will find 5% of 15. $15 \times 0.05 =$ 0.75. The answer is 0.75g.
3. 1 per cent of 200 = 2g.
4. 1:49 ratio means there are 50 parts. $50 \times 2 = 100$g. This means we must multiply both sides of the ratio by 2, giving us a ratio of 2:98. 2g + 98g = 100g. Therefore we have 2g active ingredient. The answer is 2g.
5. The cream in question 4 is stronger, as there are 2g of active ingredient in every 100g (the other cream has 2g active in every 200g, or 1g active in every 100g).

Activity 1.17 (page 32)

1. 62.5mcg = 0.0625mg
    $0.0625 \times 4 = 25$mg
    So we need 4 tablets.

2. 600mg $\times$ 2 = 1200mg = 1.2g so we need 2 doses. This means we need 2 doses $\times$ 2ml water = 4ml water.
    The answer is 4ml.

3. $\dfrac{14}{10} \times 2 = 1.4 \times 2 = 2.8$ml

    The answer is 2.8ml.

4. $\dfrac{20}{50} \times 2 = 0.8$ml

    The answer is 0.8ml.

5. 0.25 (grams) $\times$ 1000 = 250mg

    $\dfrac{250}{500} \times 5 = 2.5$ml

    The answer is 2.5ml.

6. $85 \times 2 = 170$mg every 8 hours.
    $24 \div 8 = 3$, so we need 3 doses.
    3×170mg = 510mg in 24 hours

    The answer is 510mg.

7. $\dfrac{20}{10} \times 1 = 2$ml each dose
    $24 \div 6 = 4$ doses in total.
    2ml $\times$ 4 = 8ml in 24 hours.
    The answer is 8ml.

8. $0.15g = 150mcg$
$150 \div 50 = 3$, so we need 3 doses.
The answer is 3 tablets.

9. 20 drops per ml

$$\frac{300 \times 20}{3 \times 60} = \frac{6000}{180}$$

$6000 \div 180 = 33.3$ recurring, which we round to 33dpm

The answer is 33 dpm.

10 60 drops per ml

$$\frac{500 \times 60}{2.5 \times 60} = \frac{30000}{150}$$

$30,000 \div 150 = 200$ dpm

The answer is 200 dpm.

Knowledge review

Now that you have completed the chapter, how would you rate your knowledge of the following topics?

	Good	Adequate	Poor
1. Place value			
2. Addition			
3. Subtraction			
4. Multiplication			
5. Division			
6. Decimals			
7. Converting units			
8. Strength of solutions			
9. Drug calculation formulae			
10. Drip rate calculations			

Where you're not confident in your knowledge of a topic, what will you do next?

Further reading

Haighton, J, Phillips, B, Thomas, V and Holder, D (2004) *Maths the basic skills – curriculum edition.* Cheltenham: Nelson Thornes.
An excellent resource for practising your numeracy skills.

Starkings, S and Krause, L (2010) *Passing drugs calculations tests for nursing students.* Exeter: Learning Matters.
This up-to-date text is written specifically for nursing students and covers drugs calculations in detail.

Useful websites

www.mathcentre.ac.uk Useful sections about drug calculations and general numeracy skills.

Chapter 2

The law governing medicines
Dawn Gawthorpe and Dawn L Hennefer

Draft NMC Standards for Pre-registration Nursing Education

This chapter will address the following draft competencies:

Domain: Professional values

1. All nurses must practise confidently according to *The code: standards of conduct, performance and ethics for nurses and midwives* (NMC, 2008), and other ethical and legal codes, recognising and responding appropriately to situations in day-to-day practice.
7. All nurses must practise in accordance with principles and policies at all times, keeping within the boundaries of confidentiality for people, carers and colleagues.
8. All nurses must be responsible and accountable for keeping their own knowledge and skills up-to-date through continuing professional development and life-long learning. They must use evaluation, supervision and appraisal to improve their performance and enhance the safety and quality of care and service delivery.

Domain: Communication and interpersonal skills

3. All nurses must use verbal, non-verbal and written communication to listen, recognise, interpret and record people's knowledge and understanding of their needs. They must share information with others while respecting individual rights to confidentiality.
9. All nurses must maintain accurate, clear and complete written or electronic records using the right kind of language, avoiding jargon, and use plain English so that everyone involved in the care process understands the meaning.

Domain: Nursing practice and decision making

2. All nurses must listen, recognise and respond to an individual's physical, social and psychological needs. They must then plan, deliver and evaluate technically safe, competent, person-centred care that addresses all their daily activities, in partnership with people and their carers, families and other professionals.
2.1. **Adult nurses** must safely use invasive and non-invasive procedures, technological support and pharmacological management for medical and surgical nursing practice. They must take account of individual needs and preferences as well as any existing or long term health problems.
8.1. **Adult nurses** must recognise when the complexity of clinical decisions may need specialist knowledge and expertise. They must then consult or refer accordingly.

Introduction

The administration of medicines to a patient, client or service user is an important aspect of everyday clinical practice for nurses, as we have seen in Chapter 1. The process of administering medicines to patients has been developed as a result of legal and professional regulation. This chapter will help you develop your knowledge and understanding of the law and accountability in relation to medicines management in preparation for becoming a nurse. Through scenarios and various activities throughout the chapter you will be challenged to explore what you consider a nurse should, would or could do in certain situations and the legal consequences of each action. At the same time you will also gain an awareness of your role and responsibilities when working with the other professionals.

While this book is aimed at students of adult nursing it would not be unusual to find yourself caring for an adolescent, and consideration of some of the legal implications of nursing children will be explained later in the chapter.

Legislation by and large governs our everyday lives, so that civil order can be maintained and we are kept safe. Nursing is no exception; as a profession not only do we abide by the law of the land but we also adhere to the standards and guidance set out by our regulatory body the Nursing and Midwifery Council (NMC). Generally any document that contains the word **Act** indicates it is **statute** law.

In relation to nursing and medicines, the Medicines Act (1968) and (1971) and the Misuse of Drugs Act (1971) are of great importance as they cover the licensing, supply, storage and administration of medicines.

Medicines licensing

Before a drug is granted a licence for use in the UK or Europe the pharmaceutical companies have the option of applying for a licence either directly to the Medicines and Healthcare products Regulatory Agency (MHRA) for a UK licence (or to the European Medicines Agency (EMA) for an EU licence). The MHRA will receive a dossier from the pharmaceutical company about the medicine it wishes to apply for a licence for. The application will be reviewed by an independent committee known as the Committee on Safety of Medicines (CSM), which will produce a report that will either recommend a licence, accept the application dependent on some modifications, or reject the application, giving reasons for the rejection. Licensing is based on the safety and effectiveness of the drug and the overall benefit it will have to society (Davies, 2003).

Pharmaceutical companies invest heavily in researching and developing new drugs, and running **clinical trials**, as well as production and marketing. During the drug development stages, all aspects of pharmacokinetics and pharmacodynamics are explored and the route of administration determined. The drug is then designed accordingly; for example, a protective coating (enteric coating) may be applied to a drug that is to be administered orally to protect the stomach lining from irritant ingredients. The protective coating will prevent the drug from being dissolved in the stomach by the stomach acids, but will allow the drug to be dissolved in the small intestine. Pharmaceutical companies' guidance displays all the relevant information for that drug in relation to the route to be administered, **contraindications** and side effects in the product information. The Medicines Act of 1968 was essentially initiated by the thalidomide tragedy, which was an event that occurred during the latter end of the 1950s and early 1960s. The Medicines Act made it compulsory for all medicines to be licensed before they could be introduced to the UK market.

CASE STUDY

In the late 1950s the drug thalidomide was introduced into the European market, initially marketed as a sedative. In 1957 the German pharmaceutical company Grünenthal released the drug into the German market as a sleeping pill and anti-nausea drug to treat morning sickness in pregnancy. At the same time an Australian obstetrician was prescribing this drug for his patients for antenatal use, but in the early 1960s the same obstetrician noticed that the babies born to some of the women who had taken the drug had birth defects. A paediatrician from Hamburg also made the connection between thalidomide and birth defects. After more reports were highlighted, Grünenthal withdrew the drug from the market. By 1962 the drug was banned in most countries.

CASE STUDY continued

> The case study poses us several questions to think about. How has the thalidomide tragedy affected drug prescribing in pregnancy? What is the nurse's role in advising pregnant women on what drugs they can safely take? The ethical issues associated with the continued use of thalidomide are discussed in Chapter 3.

Medicines Act (1968) and (1971) and amended directions (2000)

The Medicines Act was originally passed in 1968. It covers many different aspects of the use of medicines, ranging from animal testing to licensing.

There are three categories of drugs for public use.

- P (pharmacy medicines) are those that can be sold under the supervision of a pharmacist in a registered premises. These are medicines you would buy at a chemist without a general practitioner (GP) prescription, but that cannot be sold from a supermarket or shop.
- GSL (general sales list) are those medicines that can be sold without supervision. There are no controlled drugs on the general sales list.
- POM (prescription only medicines) are those that are sold in accordance with a prescription from an authorised prescriber. So, for example, a GP (authorised prescriber) might prescribe antibiotics that could not be bought over the counter in a chemist (unless requested by a prescription) and could certainly not be bought from the corner shop or supermarket.

The *British National Formulary* is published jointly by the British Medical Journal Group and the Royal Pharmaceutical Society of Great Britain. It is a vital reference book for nurses, doctors and other health professionals. The *BNF* contains information about all the medicines available on the National Health Service. The information it presents in relation to each medicine includes dosage, appearance, side effects and contraindications. With regard to drugs for public use, the *BNF* identifies them utilising the categories from the Medicines Act.

Activity 2.1	Evidence-based practice and research

Using a copy of the *British National Formulary* or accessing the online version (http://bnf.org/bnf/), categorise the medicines listed below into the three groups described above.

    paracetamol
    Vitamin C
    Gaviscon liquid
    Voltarol gel
    Imigran tablets
    codeine
    co-codamol
    penicillin
    diazepam

Discussion of this activity can be found at the end of the chapter.

This activity aims to help you familiarise yourself with the *British National Formulary*. By utilising the *BNF* to find the answers to this activity you can see that it is important for a nurse to develop a working knowledge of the different categories of medicines.

Activity 2.2   *Evidence-based practice and research*

Look again at the information in the *British National Formulary* on the medicine penicillin. Where do you think this information comes from?

Discussion of this activity can be found at the end of the chapter.

Because there are thousands of different medicines, you will need to access a copy of the *BNF* at every available opportunity to foster your knowledge base in order for you to administer medicines safely. The information in the *BNF* comes from the literature that a manufacturer produces as well as literature presented in pharmaceutical and medical journals and books. Information in the *BNF* can also be produced by regulatory authorities such as the National Prescribing Centre.

If we go back and think about legislation (law) that governs medicines administration, we realise that it has to be updated to ensure that patient safety is paramount. The Health Act 2006 introduced new laws on the use of controlled drugs that will be discussed in more detail later in this chapter. Since 2006 the National Prescribing Centre has updated its good practice guide (NPC, 2009a) in the management of controlled drugs within a primary care setting to help nurses practise within a legal framework.

There have been many documented incidents related to medicines errors, ranging from minor mishaps to fatalities; however, the constant factor in most of these cases is that at some stage in the process an error was made that could have been avoided. Should you find yourself involved in an incident as described below you would be asked to explain yourself. We use the term **accountability** and it is about you being asked to give an account of your actions or omissions: what you did or did not do.

Accountability

Scenario

Sheila is a registered nurse, and she is conducting a medicines round in the ward. She checks Mr Rogers' medicines (placing them in the medicines pot) and because he is not by his bed she places the medicines on his bedside locker for him to take on his return. She makes a mental note to remind him. Sheila then becomes distracted by another patient; she locks the medicines trolley and goes to attend to the patient. In the meantime Mr Daly, who is in the bed next to Mr Rogers and is disorientated, ingests Mr Rogers' medicines. When Mr Rogers returns to his bed he calls Sheila and asks for his medicines. She tells him they are on his locker, but when they investigate the medicines pot is found empty on Mr Daly's bedside locker. Mr Daly has not yet received his medicines.

Activity 2.3   *Team working*

Imagine you are the nurse in Sheila's position. Who might ask you to explain what you did in regard to the incident?

Discussion of this activity can be found at the end of the chapter.

During the first two months of 2010 the NMC disciplined a small number of nurses in relation to issues surrounding medicines administration. There are a number of sanctions and disposal open to the panel hearing the cases, and all decisions of the panel are released to employers and to the public for a period of three months. In February 2010, for example, one nurse was given a suspension order for one year for failing to demonstrate knowledge and skills in relation to insulin administration. A nurse who had failed to check a patient's name band or complete the drug round was given a caution for three years. You have to remember there are some 600,000 registrants (www.nmc-uk.org).

The activity above has introduced the idea that nurses are accountable for their actions and omissions. There are four different arenas in which nurses are accountable:

1. to the Nursing and Midwifery Council who act as a professional regulator;
2. to their employer through their employment contract;
3. to the public via civil law;
4. to society through public law.

Using these four areas of accountability as the structure for this section, we will identify a nurse's accountability in medicines management in more depth. First, you need to have an understanding of how law is classified in the UK and what each of the categories comprises. We will also look at how law is created.

Categories of law

Figure 2.1 is a diagrammatic representation of how different kinds of law are classified.

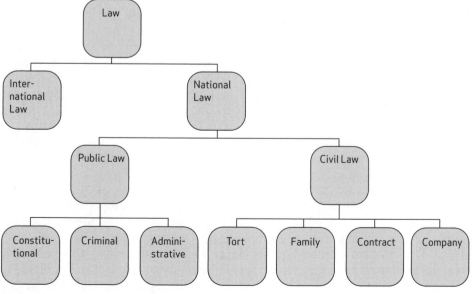

Figure 2.1 Hierarchy of law

International and national law

International law deals with issues such as who has the rights to fish around the UK coastline, whereas national law is the law that governs individual countries. Within the UK, Scotland has had its own law since devolution in 1998, while England and Wales have the same law. Northern Ireland utilises the statutes of the UK Parliament as well as some of the acts created by its own Assembly.

Public and civil (private) law

The next division in law is between public and private law (also referred to as civil law). Public law is concerned with disputes that arise in matters concerning the government or the nation. The subdivisions of this are:

- Constitutional law, which covers matters such who has the right to vote, known as suffrage;
- Administrative law, dealing with how public bodies such as the NHS should conduct themselves;
- Criminal law, which identifies types of behaviour that society deems to be illegal and the suitable punishment.

Private law occurs between businesses or private individuals. The subdivisions of this are:

- Contract law, which governs acceptable practice in relation to the buying and selling of goods;
- **Tort**, defined as a civil wrong where one person has a legal responsibility to another person – it deals with issues such as nuisance, negligence and defamation;
- Family law, which considers issues arising when parents separate or divorce as well as clarifying issues around will making and inheritance;
- Company law, regulating how businesses should be run – it includes employment law, which governs anything to do with employment such as minimum wages or holiday entitlement.

Law is made in a number of ways. The first is by **judicial precedent** where past decisions of judges (precedents) help create the law of the future. So a judge hearing a case in 2009 might utilise precedents from 1861, 1990, or from any prior case to help make a judgement. This type of law is also referred to as **case law**. Case law is reported in a number of ways; in this fictitious example, *Harry* v *Mary* [2010] 9 ALL ER 245, Harry, the **claimant**, is bringing a case against Mary, and the 'v' stands for 'versus' (against). The case was brought in the year 2010 and it can be found in Volume 9 of the *All England Law Reports*. The ER refers to Elizabeth Regina (in the reign of Queen Elizabeth) and it starts at section 245. Sometimes a **case citation** may include other initials to indicate the court it was heard in or where it was reported, so the main citation might be followed by an 'AC' for the Court of Appeal or a 'WLR' for the *Weekly Law Reports*, for example.

New laws are made by Parliament as Acts of Parliament or Statute. When the government wishes to write a new statute they follow a process that starts in the House of Commons with the drafting of a Bill; this Bill undergoes two readings in the House of Commons before passing through a committee and reporting stage where all parliamentary parties are represented. The aim of these various readings is to make any necessary amendments before it returns for a third reading in the House of Commons. The Bill then goes to the House of Lords where the whole procedure is repeated and finally it gains **royal assent** and the Bill is entered onto the Statute book to become law.

The Supreme Court of the United Kingdom deals with appeals from the most complex cases, related predominantly to judicial reviews. Judgements can be made by the court or by separate judges, who are called Justices of the Supreme Court.

It is important that nurses who administer medication do not find themselves liable for **trespass to the person** under the Offences against the Person Act 1861 through a charge of assault and/or battery.

Activity 2.4   *Critical thinking*

In this chapter only a brief summary of a legal case will be presented. You can access original case or Statute Law at most University and College libraries, which have access to an electronic legal database or paper sources such as *The All England Law Reports* or *The Law Reports*. There are numerous textbooks on law, some specifically on law and nursing practice (see Further reading at the end of this chapter). Information on Acts of Parliament can be found on the Office of Public Sector Information website at www.opsi.gov.uk.

In order to fully understand the decisions made in the cases presented, you should try to access one of the databases identified, and using the help functions, see if you can find the full text of the case. To start with, access the Office of Public Sector Information (OPSI) and see if you can find the Equality Act 2010. If you are unfamiliar with using databases, then as part of your ongoing professional development, make an appointment with the librarian at your institute to find out if study skills sessions are offered.

As this is an activity to develop your research skills, there is no answer at the end of the chapter.

All nurses must gain their patient's **consent** before any intervention, and medicines administration is no exception. Competent patients have a right to self-determination that is established in law in cases such as *Schloendorff* v *Society of New York Hospitals* [1914]. This identifies the legal position of consent in the fact that a person and only that person can decide what will happen to them. In terms of medicines management, this means that it is the patient who can decide whether to accept or decline medicines. The next issue that can arise is where someone else questions the choice the person has made. The case of Re T (*Adult Refusal of Treatment* [1992] 3 WLR clarifies that every person is presumed to have capacity to consent unless it is proven otherwise, and it defines the legal position on testing capacity. A person lacking capacity to consent can be treated in their best interests as set out in *F* v *West Berkshire Health Authority* [1990].

So now that we have seen where laws come from, let us explore each of these arenas of accountability in turn.

Accountability to the NMC

The Nursing and Midwifery Order 2001 (SI 2003/253) established the Nursing and Midwifery Council in 2002. The NMC's primary purpose is to ensure that its registrants (registered nurses) provide a high quality of safe care. It aims to promote these standards through the production of guidance for both its registrants and its student nurses on what it considers to be professional conduct in publications such as *The Code* (p40). The NMC provides advice and considers allegations of misconduct or incompetence against its members, as well as unfitness to practise, so if your fitness to practise is questioned in relation to any aspect of medicines management, you may well find yourself having to explain your actions or omissions to an NMC panel.

Scenario

Mr Daly, the patient in the earlier scenario, has missed his medicines again. The scenario this time is slightly different.

Sheila, the registered nurse, checks Mr Rogers' medicines (placing them in the medicines pot) and because he is not by his bed she puts the medicines on the bedside locker for him to take on his return. Another nurse, Margaret, is leaning against a locker belonging to a Mr Graham, which is the locker next to the one used by Mr Daly. Sheila places the tablets on the locker as before, saying 'They are for him'. Margaret assumes the tablets are for her patient, Mr Graham. Margaret picks up the medicine pot and gives the tablets to Mr Graham who happily takes them.

What might happen to Sheila and Margaret in terms of accountability to the NMC? If the nurses' employers feel that these actions were serious enough, they can be referred to the NMC directly. The NMC has a number of fitness to practise panels and the case would be referred to the investigating committee first. They would want to know how the drug was given to the wrong patient. They would require an explanation of why the nurses deviated from the advice given in their own *Standards for medicines management*. If they considered the actions and/or omissions of these two nurses constituted professional misconduct, the case would be forwarded to that committee panel.

In relation to medicines management there are numerous systems in place within the care environments in the form of policies, guidance and procedures to maintain the safety of both patients and staff. However, given human nature, differences of opinion can arise between co-workers, and how this is managed is important. If you feel uncomfortable with the prescription presented to you, you must question the prescriber or pharmacist and give a sound rationale for your difference of opinion. If you foster good working relationships with other colleagues within the clinical area, they will help you and offer you support. This aspect of multidisciplinary working will be discussed further in Chapter 6.

Accountability to your employer

The second arena of accountability is to your employer, which is a category of civil law. Within this field of law **vicarious liability** comes into play. Vicarious liability is the liability an employer accepts for any acts that their staff may commit. This is on the proviso that the practitioner has practised in accordance with company policy and guidance, and also within the law.

Nurses have a professional duty to notify their employer if they feel that a company policy does not meet legal requirements. As long as an employee practises within these reasonable instructions or legal requirements, the employer accepts liability. Where a nurse does make a mistake, the employer has the right to instigate its own disciplinary process, but consideration of the nurse's honesty and actions to minimise further harm to the patient will be a factor in the decision made.

If a nurse is dismissed, then under the Employment Act 2002 they have the right of appeal. Patients do in certain cases choose to make a claim against individual nurses and, as the employee, you could be found liable; however, the claimant has to prove that the person who carried out the negligent act was an employee at the time.

Professional accountability

We have considered your accountability as an individual in relation to your own practice as a nurse, but we also need to explore what accountability you have towards fellow nurses. One area of anxiety for students and registered nurses alike is what to do when they have concerns about the behaviour of a nursing colleague.

If a nurse finds a colleague misusing drugs, for example, then they have a legal obligation and professional duty to report this to their manager. Should the manager fail to act upon the information provided by the concerned nurse, then the Public Interest Disclosure Act 1999 protects the nurse from victimisation should they wish to disclose this wider. The nurse should, however, familiarise herself or himself with the legal processes associated with this Act so as not to breach confidentiality.

We have now looked at two arenas of accountability and it is important to recognise here how you as a nurse might be accountable in a way that is different from some of your family or friends who are not nurses and who may feel they are accountable only to their employer. Your friends and family are, however, accountable in the two areas that we will discuss next.

Accountability to the private citizen (civil law) and to society (public law)

The final two arenas of accountability are better considered together. Civil law relates to law where an individual believes their rights have been infringed. It is sometimes called private law. The nurse can be called to account in the civil arena where a patient, relative or their representative brings a claim under the tort of negligence.

In terms of clinical negligence, the fault caused can be defined in law in two ways. First, negligence can be civil, where an action in the courts seeks to redress any harm caused by awarding monetary compensation. Second, in more serious cases, negligence can be a **criminal action**, brought through public law leading to prosecution. If one of your family and friends commits a traffic offence, they too could be found liable in civil and criminal law. So civil and criminal law affects all citizens of the UK and we are all accountable in law. Before we discuss your accountability as a nurse under civil and public law, it is useful to have an overview of the differences in terms of how the courts deal with cases.

Table 2.1 sets out the differences between cases brought under civil law in comparison to criminal law cases.

Table 2.1: Civil and criminal cases compared

	Civil case	Criminal case
What the law seeks to do	Uphold individual rights	Protect societal values
Who brings the case?	The individual known as the claimant	Crown Prosecution Service through the police by a prosecutor
In which court is the case heard?	Usually a county court or High Court	Usually at a Magistrates Court or Crown Court
Standard of proof	On the balance of probability	Beyond reasonable doubt
Who makes the decision?	Judge	Magistrate or jury
What is the decision/verdict?	Liable or not liable	Guilty or not guilty
Remedy of the court	Award of damages	Imposition of a fine, community service, prison sentence or discharge

---

Scenario

Jane is the staff nurse on Ward 21. While working a night duty shift she says she administered Mr Thomas's antibiotics at 10 p.m. and when she checked on him at midnight he was fast asleep. At 2 a.m. Mr Thomas is found unresponsive by another staff nurse and is subsequently admitted to the intensive care unit following an anaphylactic reaction. When the family are informed about the incident they are very angry and accuse Jane of being negligent.

If a patient suffers harm as a result of negligence by either the prescriber or the administrator – or both – then the patient or their next of kin or executor can bring an action. So, for example, if a patient is prescribed and administered a drug with little explanation of what the drug is for, and if the patient suffers side effects that cause harm, the law on consent could play an important part because it could be argued that the patient did not give valid consent.

Nursing is a 24-hour, seven-days-a-week activity, and care does not stop just because it is late in the night. However, part of your caring role as a nurse is to try to ensure that where clinical assessment allows it, patients are given the opportunity to rest. In the scenario presented here, the aim might be to ensure that Mr Thomas gets a good night's sleep. What is being questioned is what caused the harm to Mr Thomas and whether Jane should have done something to prevent the harm or whether she did something that caused the harm. Would other nurses in a similar position have left Mr Thomas to sleep? What needs to be established is whether Jane did what she should have done. If you put yourself in Jane's position, what would you have done? This allows you to consider the difficulties faced when trying to decide if someone has been negligent or not.

Another example might be a situation where a patient refuses to take a medicine and, as a result of this refusal, their condition deteriorates and they die. The family may bring a claim in negligence because they feel that you as the nurse should have done more to ensure their relative took the medicine. Here again, the issue of the right of a patient to consent to or refuse treatment would be important in determining liability, as the patient may have decided not to take the medicine, having been informed of all the side effects.

Negligence

Negligence is legally defined in the case of Anderson B in *Blyth v Birmingham Waterworks Co* (1856) 11EXCH 781 as: *the omission to do something which a reasonable man, guided upon those considerations which ordinarily regulate the conduct of human affairs, would do, or doing something which a prudent and reasonable man would not do.* In a different and more recent case Lord Justice Wright in *Lochgelly v McMullan* [1934] AC1.25 stated, *this means more than heedless or careless conduct, whether in omission or commission: it properly connotes the complex concept of duty, breach and damage thereby suffered by the person to whom the duty was owing.*

We can see from both these legal definitions that there is more than one thing to be considered and proven for someone to be negligent. There are four elements that the patient (claimant) has to prove to succeed in a claim of negligence. These are:

1. that the **defendant** owed a duty of care to the person harmed (duty);
2. that they breached that duty (breach);
3. that the breach caused was foreseeable (causation);
4. that there was harm caused to the claimant (harm).

Often they are more simply referred to as duty, breach, causation and harm. So should a patient, relative or representative wish to make a claim for negligence against you as the nurse, you need to be familiar with these to attempt to reduce that risk. Each of the elements will be considered in turn.

Duty of care

Nurses have a 'duty of care', which means they must act in the best interests of their patients, acknowledge their limitations in relation to both knowledge and skill, and ensure that no act or omission of theirs should be injurious to patients.

Duty of care was defined by Lord Atkin when he gave judgement in the case of *Donoghue v Stephenson* (House of Lords) (1932), cited in NMC 2008. He stated:

> You must take reasonable care to avoid acts or omissions which you can reasonably foresee would be likely to injure your neighbour. Who, then, in the law is my neighbour? The answer seems to be persons who are so closely and directly affected by my act that I ought to have them in contemplation as being so affected when I am directing my mind to the acts or omissions which are called in question.

CASE STUDY

A nurse–patient relationship is a 'duty situation' as recognised in *Kent* v *Griffiths and Others* [2000] 2ALL ER 474.

The 'Griffiths' in this case was a pregnant lady. While at home she suffered an asthma attack. Her GP called for an ambulance and when it didn't arrive he called again. The ambulance arrived after 40 minutes, taking some 26 minutes longer than the time stipulated in the ambulance service's own guidelines at the time. Even though Griffiths was given oxygen on the way to the hospital she suffered a respiratory arrest, was brain damaged and miscarried. She brought a case against the ambulance service.

Do you think there is a liability in negligence here?

This lady was awarded £95,000 because the ambulance service was found to be liable. This was because they were considered a health service, unlike other emergency services. Nursing is also a health service, so we always owe our patients a duty of care that spans all aspects of practice, including medicines management. Part of your duty of care in relation to medicines administration is always to seek consent from an adult with capacity, and if the patient is without capacity, you are required to act in the best interest of that patient. The relatively new Mental Capacity Act (2005) also recognises a duty of care; in Section 42 it creates the offence of ill treatment or neglect of a person lacking capacity by anyone responsible for that person's care.

So how can you be sure that you have discharged your duty of care?

Legally, this has been defined in two cases, often referred to simply as the Bolam and the Bolitho tests.

Bolam v Friern Hospital Management Committee [1957] 1 W.L.R.582

Mr Bolam was a voluntary patient at a psychiatric unit run by the Friern Hospital Management Committee. While a patient there he consented to undergo electro-convulsive therapy (ECT). He was not given any relaxant drugs, and his body was not restrained during the procedure. During the procedure he had an ECT-induced seizure during which he suffered fractures. He brought a claim in negligence against the hospital suggesting that they were negligent for not prescribing and giving him muscle relaxants, not restraining him and not warning him about the risks involved.

The Bolam case set a precedent that has become known as the Bolam test that identifies the standard of care that practitioners can be measured against.

Judge McNair stated that the test is the standard of *the ordinary skilled man exercising and professing to have that skill . . . it is sufficient if he exercises the ordinary skill of an ordinary competent man exercising that particular art. [A doctor] is not guilty of negligence if he has acted in accordance with a practice accepted as proper by a responsible body of medical men skilled in that particular art.*

Bolitho v City and Hackney HA [1997] 4 ALL ER 771

Patrick Bolitho, a two-year-old boy, suffered brain damage when a paediatric registrar failed to attend to him. The boy had developed respiratory problems but then improved slightly on two occasions during the same afternoon. The ward sister was concerned and called the doctor on both occasions and even asked another nurse to sit with the patient. On the third occasion in the same afternoon the boy's condition deteriorated rapidly and his respiratory failure led to a cardiac arrest. Although he was revived, he had been without oxygen for a considerable amount of time, leading to brain damage, and he died some time later. The case centred on whether or not intubating the patient might have made a difference to the outcome.

One side argued that had the registrar attended, the child would not have been intubated while the opposing side argued about the registrar's failure to intubate, saying this was reasonable behaviour. The judgement stated that medical practitioners must not escape liability even where all the experts agree and where the evidence for both sides has a logical basis. The judgement was that not intubating was not a negligent act, even though the **expert opinion** was divided.

Duty and breach

We have already explained about duty of care; in the case of a person claiming negligence, we have identified that the claimant (person who is claiming) must prove that the nurse had a duty of care towards them and that in exercising that duty of care it was breached in some way. Once this is established, it is necessary to explore if the breach could have been prevented, which leads us to causation.

We can apply this to the scenario about Jane the staff nurse (on page 50) who had a duty of care to her patient. Jane also had a duty to consider if there were any reasons why she should not have administered the antibiotic in the first place, such as checking that the patient had no allergies. In considering whether there was a breach of that duty, the judge would seek advice from nurse experts and utilise the *Standards for medicines management* document as well as any local policies from the hospital where Jane worked to determine what would be the reasonable and acceptable standard, as set in the Bolam and Bolitho cases.

Causation

Causation is the next element that would need to be proved for a successful claim in negligence. The following two cases seek to demonstrate the complexities of proving causation.

Kay v Ayrshire and Arran Health Board [1987] 2ALL ER 417

A child suffering with meningitis was administered 300,000 units of penicillin instead of 10,000. The child became deaf following the administration of the drug. What needed to be established was **causation** – could a link be established between the amount of drug administered and the harm suffered? Meningitis itself can cause deafness. The case was heard in a number of courts after the judge found for the claimants (parents). The parents claimed that it was the over-dosage that had caused the deafness. However, when the case was heard in the House of Lords, the discussion centred on the fact that there were two potential causes of the damage and they rejected the parents' claim for factual causation. It needed to be proved that it was the over-dosage that caused the deafness and it could not be.

Wilsher v Essex Health Authority CA.1986 3.All, ER 801 HL 1988 1 ALL ER 871

Martin Wilsher was born three months premature. He was admitted to the Special Care Baby Unit (SCBU) on oxygen therapy via a face mask. While on the SCBU a junior doctor mistakenly inserted a catheter into an umbilical vein for arterial blood gas sampling. The error was missed by both a senior registrar and a consultant radiologist. When the catheter was changed, it was again placed into an umbilical vein instead of the artery. As a result of this Martin Wilsher was given an overdose of oxygen and he developed retrolental fibroplasia, a condition that caused severe damage to his eyesight. The Court of Appeal dismissed an appeal by the health authority because the judge was so concerned that *a health authority which so conducts its hospital that it fails to provide doctors of sufficient skill and experience to give the treatment offered at the hospital may be directly liable in negligence to the patient.* The judge awarded damages of £116,199.

Activity 2.6   *Critical thinking*

This is a brief description of a case where a patient was left brain damaged as a result of a drug error.

Prendergast v Sam & Dee [1988] (case 11)

In 1983 Mr Prendergast obtained a prescription from his GP for a number of items including a course of amoxil (an antibacterial drug). Mr Kozary, the pharmacist at Sam & Dee Ltd, dispensed all of the items correctly apart from the amoxil. Mr Kozary dispensed Daonil instead, which was a brand name for glibenclamide (a hypoglycaemic agent) at the time of the case.

Identify who you think is liable, and why.

Discussion of this activity can be found at the end of the chapter.

Record keeping

Good record keeping is essential in providing care. Not only does it identify how, where, when and to whom you provide your care but it also identifies the assessments you made, the decision-making processes involved and whether the care you delivered was effective or not. How you keep your records will depend on your employer; whether they are handwritten or electronic the same principles apply. In terms of the law, your records are your proof of what has occurred: if it is not documented, then it did not happen. It is essential, therefore, that you take great care when documenting hospital in-patients' records, because if a patient makes a claim, by the time the case is heard you may well have difficulty remembering the actual events that led to the incident and so your documentation could be your defence. Usually, more than one person is involved in medicines administration. As a nurse you might be the administrator who gives the patient their medicines, but the medicines will have been prescribed by someone else and the pharmacist may have been involved in the checking and dispensing of the prescription. Good record keeping is useful when trying to look back and provide a paper trail of a series of events.

To remind yourself of the principles of record keeping, look in the Further reading section at the end of this chapter.

Harm

We have considered both duty of care and breach of a duty of care, and we have seen how causation can be established. The next element to a successful claim is that of harm.

One area of concern for nurses is the situation where a patient cannot take a medicine in a certain form, such as when a patient has difficulty swallowing and has been dispensed tablets. If you were nursing that patient, you might well mix the tablets with a liquid such as water or crush them into a powder but there are legal implications for such practice.

Crushing medicines

When drugs are crushed it is usually with the best intentions for the patient. However, you as a student nurse need to be aware of the implications of crushing medicines. First, it can potentially alter the therapeutic properties of a drug, as discussed in Chapter 4. A patient could be harmed as a result. If a drug is licensed for use with a protective coating that is then breached by crushing, the nurse will be administering the drug in an unlicensed form.

If you feel your patient cannot swallow tablets, you as the nurse should always consult with the prescriber or pharmacist to explore if a drug could be given in a different format.

At the start of the chapter we outlined how a case brought in civil law has the legal remedy of compensation for the harm caused. Under the Civil Liability Contribution Act 1978 the claimant may bring a case against more than one defendant. The following case demonstrates how liability is decided.

Dwyer v Roderick [1984] QBD

Dr Roderick prescribed the drug Migril (for the treatment of acute migraine) for Mrs Dwyer. Mrs Dwyer also saw another GP, Dr Jackson, around the same time. It was claimed that the dose and frequency were incorrect and she suffered harm as a result of an overdose. This overdose led to the side effect of vasoconstriction and the development of gangrene in her toes. The tablets were dispensed from a local pharmacy where two pharmacists were on duty. Neither pharmacist noticed the error in the prescription. So who was liable?

The courts held them all liable. Mrs Dwyer was awarded £92,000 damages, but this was distributed between those found liable and their degree of liability was assessed as Dr Roderick 45 per cent, Dr Jackson 15 per cent and the two pharmacists 40 per cent.

The last element to a successful claim is that harm has been caused, and this appears clear in the case of Mrs Dwyer as she developed gangrene. What has to be proven is, was the harm a consequence of something else or was it directly related to the defendants' actions or omissions?

Interestingly, not all harm is compensatable. Grief alone is not a ground for a claim but there is a statutory right for compensation for bereavement where death resulted from negligence.

Alcock v Chief Constable South Yorkshire Police [1992] 2 AC 310HL

Shortly before the commencement of a major football match on 15 April 1989 at Hillsborough football stadium the police responsible for crowd control at the match allowed extra spectators into an already full ground, with the result that 95 spectators were crushed to death. Scenes were broadcast live on television. Sixteen persons, all of whom were relatives, brought actions against the Chief Constable, claiming damages for nervous shock. The judge found in favour of only ten of the claimants. The decision was based on the fact that as well as being closely related to the victims, these ten people were present in the ground when the tragedy occurred, whereas the others had only seen it on television and were therefore not considered to have suffered nervous shock, which was defined as a sudden assault on the nervous system.

Product liability

As well as liability of the healthcare professionals and the employers, the manufacturers of a drug, distributers, suppliers and those who sell the drug can be held liable under the area of law known as product liability. The same legal principles apply; the patient has to show that the manufacturer in this case had failed to ensure that the drug was safe in relation to its design, the way it was marketed and its information leaflets. Some of the difficulties in securing a successful claim are around whether the injuries occurred as a result of the disease process rather than the actual medicine. All drugs have side effects, and in some cases side effects are unknown despite extensive licensing, so the MHRA, mentioned earlier in the chapter, has a system called black triangle monitoring, which is ongoing surveillance of new products. Such products are marked with a black triangle in the *BNF*, showing that surveillance should be maintained. It is also sometimes difficult to get product information related to clinical trials because that information is confidential to the pharmaceutical company. The Consumer Protection Act of 1987 covers product liability, consumer safety and pricing issues, and as a number of medicines used in this country are produced elsewhere in the world, this Act extends its powers to incorporate importers. The patient could make a claim under the Sales of Goods Act (1979), which states that a product has to be fit for purpose.

CASE STUDY: *Roe v Minister of Health 1954 2QB 66*

In 1947 the claimants underwent surgery at the Chesterfield and North Derbyshire Royal Hospital. Each claimant had a spinal anaesthetic. The anaesthetic had been stored in glass ampoules that were, prior to use, immersed in a phenol solution. After their operations the claimants developed paraplegia. The injuries to the claimants were found to be caused by the anaesthetic being contaminated by the phenol through invisible cracks in the ampoules. Utilising the Bolam test, the judge said that the anaesthetists could not have been negligent because they had followed the standard practice. The risk of contamination had been unknown at the time and the situation could not be looked at using hindsight; if the risk was not known at the time then there could be no negligence.

For you as the nurse any concerns relating to any medicine must be reported using specific reporting mechanisms which will be discussed in more detail in Chapter 5. Where a specific side effect is identified, the government can amend legislation to recognise a need to compensate individuals for particular harm. An example of this is the NHS immunisation programmes. Under the **Statutory Instrument** 2002 No. 1592 The Regulatory Reform (Vaccine Damage Payments Act 1979) Order 2002, damages of £10,000 can be paid to a claimant if they are disabled as a result of vaccination against certain diseases such as tetanus.

In terms of civil law we have explored some of the complexities of how a claim might be brought and have considered the required elements for a successful claim. In civil law the remedy is compensation for the harm caused, but how does one decide how much compensation a claimant, is entitled to? In terms of the amount of monetary compensation awarded to the claimant, this relates to the claimant being in the same position as if the negligent act had not occurred. This compensation is termed **damages**. Most claims are for personal injury and the money awarded is set in a tariff that is known as **quantum**. Damages can be awarded for the pain and suffering caused, and are referred to as general damages. Another type of damages, special damages, are awarded for the expenses incurred such as healthcare costs or for future loss of earnings. Damages can be reduced in cases of contributory negligence where the person is partly to blame.

Having considered how a claim can be brought, we need to consider how you as a nurse might provide a defence.

Defences to a claim in negligence

There are four defences that can be made against a claim in negligence.

1. Denial of the facts: the defence claims that they were not to blame; remember the burden of proof is with the claimant.
2. Missing elements: one or more of the four elements (duty, breach, causation and harm) are missing.
3. *Volenti Non Fit Injuria* (to a willing person, no injury is done): an example would be people engaged in contact sports such as boxing or judo who give their consent to fight and are well aware of the risks – they would not consent to being hit by anyone in any other circumstances. They are aware of the risk and they waive their right to make a claim.
4. Contributory negligence: the claimant still has some liability and the damages awarded can be reduced. An example would be not wearing a seatbelt and claiming for personal injury in a car crash.

Limitation Act

A claimant has only a limited time span in which to bring a claim; the rules are laid out in the Limitation Act 1980. In cases of personal injury it is limited to three years; there are exceptions to these rules in cases of mental incapacity and children.

The final arena of accountability and the one which can have the most serious consequences for a nurse is accountability to society.

Criminal law

Criminal law seeks to protect individuals and society from harming themselves by providing guidance on how to behave. There are some exceptions from liability but these relate to children under the age of ten, some people detained under the Mental Health Act 1983 and those who lack capacity.

In criminal law two legal terms are used: *mens rea,* meaning the mental element of the crime, and *actus rea,* the act itself. If a patient is harmed as a result of an error relating to medicines administration and if this harm is extreme and the patient dies as a consequence of such an error, then you as the nurse could find yourself facing criminal charges for gross negligence and this could lead to a charge of manslaughter or even murder.

CASE STUDY

Beverly Allitt qualified as an enrolled nurse and secured a job at the Grantham and Kesteven General Hospital in 1991. During a three-month period she killed four children and injured nine others by administering lethal doses of potassium chloride, causing cardiac arrests, and lethal does of insulin to cause lethal hypoglycaemia.

In 1993 she was found guilty of murder and attempted murder. The court sentenced her to 13 concurrent life sentences. It was the diligence of two paediatricians who were concerned at the number of cardiac arrests on one of their wards that led to the investigation and subsequent conviction.

Using this case study we will examine how a nurse can be accountable under criminal law. An independent inquiry into the actions of Beverley Allitt case saw the publication of the Clothier Report in 1994, which recommended that at least two Registered Sick Children's Nurses (RSCN) should work each shift in a paediatric setting to reduce the risk of a nurse working alone and particularly having frequent unchecked access to the medicine cabinet.

The difference between voluntary and involuntary manslaughter

Any person who intentionally kills another may be prosecuted for murder or manslaughter (Montgomery, 2003, p464). There are two categories of manslaughter. **Voluntary manslaughter** is where the defendant has the *mens rea:* they either intended to kill or they did not consider that their actions could lead to death. **Involuntary manslaughter** is where there is no *mens rea:* the defendant did not set out to kill but the victim was severely harmed and here we use the term gross negligence.

Criminal proceedings

Following the death of a patient the coroner has to be notified in accordance with the Coroners and Justice Act 2009 Ch 25 in certain circumstances. The next activity will help familiarise you with these requirements.

Activity 2.7   *Evidence-based practice and research*

Using the website www.courtroomadvice.co.uk, answer the following questions.

- Which deaths have to be reported to a coroner?
- What are the possible findings of a Coroner's Court?
- What proceedings may follow a coroner's inquest?

Discussion of this activity can be found at the end of the chapter.

Controlled drugs

Dame Janet Smith led the inquiry into the conduct of the former doctor Harold Shipman, who was found guilty of murdering some of his patients by abusing his position as a GP. Shipman was convicted in January 2000 of the murders of 15 of his patients. It is believed he told them that they were being given vitamin injections or that a blood sample was being taken, when in reality he was giving them lethal doses of morphine. As a consequence of this, each hospital trust must now have an accountable officer whose role is to take responsibility for the safe use of controlled drugs. Controlled drugs are discussed further in Chapter 5.

Medicines administration and children

In English law consent is required before treatment begins. In the case of children under the age of 18 this also applies, but in what appears as a more complex way.

The Family Law Reform Act 1969 Sec 8(1) allows children who have attained 16 years of age to consent on their own behalf for surgical, medical or dental treatment, including the administration of an anaesthetic. For some parents it might seem disconcerting that a child can consent to something quite serious without them knowing, and in 1985 Mrs Victoria Gillick brought just such a case, *Gillick v West Norfolk and Wisbech Area Health Authority and another* [1985] 2 BMLR 11. Mrs Gillick challenged whether or not girls under 16 could consent to contraceptive advice. Mrs Gillick was concerned that allowing under-16s to gain advice without parental consent might be encouraging young people to commit a criminal offence under the Sexual Offences Act of 1967 (which was replaced in 2003 by the current Act), and also have a damaging effect on society as a whole.

There were two outcomes from this case. The first has become known as Gillick Competence and states that in certain circumstances a child under 16 has the capacity to give their own consent, which will be regarded as legally valid if they fulfil certain criteria: they have the intellectual emotional and maturity as well as the ability to understand what the proposed treatment is. The second outcome is the Fraser Guidelines, which specifically relates to contraceptive advice and treatment to under-16s. The Fraser Guidelines are clear in their advice that any healthcare professional should:

> believe the girl or boy understands the advice and cannot be persuaded to include the parents and that there is concern that the person will continue to engage in sexual intercourse without contraception. If we consider the best interest of the person then the health care professional has an obligation to provide advice treatment or both.

C H A P T E R   S U M M A R Y

This aims of this chapter have been to simplify some of the more complex issues surrounding legislation and its interpretation with regard to medicines management. The categorisation of law itself is complicated, and an attempt has been made to demonstrate where you as the student nurse may be involved and how you can be accountable. Remember you are accountable in four different arenas: the regulatory body; your employer; the public; and society as a whole. You have a duty of care to your patient by promoting their best interests at all times. Any breach of this duty could result in you being called to account for your actions or omissions. Medicines and its management is only one aspect of care delivery. It is important to remember that the support of registrants, educationalists, medical staff and pharmacists and your own vigilance will help to minimise medicines errors. It is important to remember that when you are qualified, it is a regulatory requirement for you to both acknowledge your limitations and develop your knowledge and skills in relation to the legal and professional requirements of medicines management.

Activities: brief outline answers

Activity 2.1: Evidence-based practice and research (page 43)

Feeling scared about the responsibilities of medicines administration is not unusual; a number of student nurses wonder how they will ever remember all the names of medicines and what they are prescribed for. Using the *BNF* or specific product information leaflets will aid your knowledge development about categories of other medicines. So when we look up paracetamol we find that it is in both the GSL and pharmacy categories and when combined with other medicines it can be a prescription only medicine.

Activity 2.2: Evidence-based practice and research (page 44)

Information relating to the medicine penicillin can also be found in the *BNF* or in the product information leaflet. The information provided tells you about the indications for use, any cautions that might be associated with this particular medicine and its potential side effects. Suggested doses are also described. Particularly with penicillin, referred to as anti-bactericidal medicine, to avoid the development of resistance the prescriber is advised to refer to any National Institute for Health and Clinical Excellence (NICE) Guidelines or local policy guidance in respect of their use in different clinical settings. The cost of the medicine is given as well as the different forms in which it can be prescribed, such as oral solution or injection.

As a particular medicine may be manufactured by more than one company, the *BNF* also provides a description of the product in terms of colour and markings.

The prescriber is advised to check that the patient does not have an allergy to this particular medicine as they could develop an anaphylactic reaction, which could be fatal.

There is a product leaflet included within the packaging of a medicine; for example, penicillin tablets are usually supplied either in a medicine bottle or in blister packs and there will always be a product leaflet included for the patient to take away with them.

Activity 2.3: Team working (page 45)

The patient himself or a relative of Mr Daly might want an explanation because they might be anxious about the potential harmful effects resulting from this error. They might wish to complain about Sheila's actions, and the nurse manager might instigate an investigation and therefore also require an account of the events. As a result of this investigation Sheila might be asked to present her account to her employer as part of a disciplinary process. The matter could also be referred to the NMC if anyone considers that Sheila is not fit to practise as a nurse and this would be dealt with by disciplinary committee panels. If physical or psychological harm was caused to Mr Daly, his family might wish to sue the nurse and they might seek compensation or a criminal conviction. So Sheila might be asked to explain the circumstances in a court of law.

Activity 2.5: Critical thinking (page 49)

Activity 2.5 is about how the nurse can be accountable through her employment contract. In relation to pay, an employer has a duty to pay an employee wages, which gives the employee the right to claim against the employer if they are unpaid, and while the employee is in paid employment the employee has a duty to obey reasonable orders. In relation to nursing, these orders could be following trust policies with regard to the administration of medicines or the storage of drugs, for example, the requirement to keep controlled drugs locked in a cupboard within a cupboard. If a nurse contravenes this requirement they are in breach of their contract and the employer has the right to dismiss the employee for misconduct.

All employers have a duty to provide a safe system of work for their employees, who could make a claim if they are injured as a result of an unsafe system; this places a duty on the nurse to report any breaches of this system to the employer. For example, if the employee is expected to administer chemotherapy agents, then the employer is required to provide the correct safety equipment for staff.

How do you think a person might find out where a nurse works? The NMC has a facility whereby anyone can search the register to find out the geographical area in which someone works but not the actual place of work.

The employer is accountable to the employee to make them aware of the policies and procedures that should govern their practice. It is common for many Trusts and PCTs (Primary Care Trusts) to use the intranet to ensure staff are made aware of any updates or changes in local policy with regard to medicine administration. The obligation for the employee is to keep themselves updated.

Activity 2.6: Critical thinking (page 54)
In this case study the arguments centred on the illegible handwriting of the doctor and the pharmacist's failure to pick up on the massive discrepancy in drug dosage – the glibenclamide came in 5mg tablets and the prescription was for 250mg. The pharmacist should have recognised and questioned what appeared to be a massive dose. The other issue was to establish who was negligent – the doctor, the pharmacist, or both. The blame was apportioned as 75 per cent to the pharmacist and 25 per cent to the doctor. As a nurse, if you are in any doubt about the legibility of a prescription, you have a duty to ask the prescriber to come and write it more legibly. You should also ensure that your own handwriting is always legible.

Activity 2.7: Evidence-based practice and research (page 58)
In all cases where the cause of death is unknown the coroner has to be informed. Other examples are where the deceased died a violent or unnatural death, the death was caused by a notifiable accident, poisoning or disease, or the deceased died while in custody. The coroner can make one of a number of findings. There are short findings such as accident, misadventure, drug related, and natural causes; where there is no clear cause of death, an open verdict may be given.

Knowledge review

Now that you have completed the chapter, how would you rate your knowledge of the following topics? Remember that the knowledge you have gained should be commensurate with the expectation of the NMC proficiencies.

	Good	Adequate	Poor
1. The four areas where a nurse can be called to be accountable			
2. How the law is organised in the UK			
3. The legal framework in relation to medicines management			

Where you're not confident in your knowledge of a topic, what will you do next?

Further reading

Dimond, B (2008) *Legal aspects of nursing*, 5th edition. Harlow: Pearson Education. A very useful introductory text for student nurses that comprehensibly covers many aspects relating to nursing practice.

Griffith, R and Tengnah, C (2010) *Law and professional issues in nursing.* Exeter: Learning Matters.

Hodgson, J (2010) The UK's Supreme Court: how it works and why it exists. *British Journal of Nursing* 18 (3).
An article giving information about the recent developments in the judicial system in the UK. This will help you in understanding the process that a claimant might have to undergo.

Montgomery, J (2003) *Health care law,* 2nd edition. New York: Oxford University Press.
A more technical legal textbook that offers more in depth analysis of cases pertaining to healthcare practice in the wider context.

Nursing and Midwifery Council (2010) *Record keeping: guidance for nurses and midwives,* London: NMC.
As a student you should access and download a copy of the NMC's guidance on record keeping to familiarise yourself with the legal, professional and ethical obligations of nurses in relation to record keeping.

Useful websites

www.contergan.grunenthal.info Allows you to read in more detail about the issues surrounding the complications of the medicine thalidomide.

www.mhra.gov.uk Concerned with the regulation of medicines.

www.opsi.gov.uk Publishes statutes.

Chapter 3

Ethical frameworks

Dawn Gawthorpe

Draft NMC Standards for Pre-registration Nursing Education

This chapter will address the following draft competencies:

Domain: Professional values

Graduate nurses must show professionalism, integrity and caring by working in partnership with people and their carers and other health and social care professionals and agencies, within professional, ethical and legal frameworks.

Draft Essential Skills Clusters

This chapter will address the following draft ESCs:

Cluster: Medicines management

34. People can trust the newly registered graduate nurse to work within legal and ethical frameworks that underpin safe and effective medicines management.

By the second progression point:

i. Demonstrates understanding of legal and ethical frameworks relating to the safe administration of medicines in practice

By entry to the register:

iv. Applies legislation to practice to safe and effective ordering, receiving, storing administering and disposal of medicines and drugs, including controlled drugs in both primary and secondary care settings and ensures others do the same.

Chapter aims

After reading this chapter, you will be able to:

* explain the terms 'ethics' and 'morals';
* describe two ethical theories that might be used in decision making;

Chapter aims continued

- recognise situations where you can be called to account for your actions and omissions in relation to medicines management;
- consider the ethical dilemmas faced by adult nurses when participating in medicines management in a variety of clinical settings.

Introduction

Medicines administration can be regarded as one of the most common therapeutic interventions undertaken in the National Health Service (NHS). In 2001, the Audit Commission suggested that about 7,000 doses were administered daily in a typical hospital. No matter what the medicine is prescribed for, no one drug can be described as being 100 per cent safe. The very nature of medicines is that they change or alter a physiological response in the body. All drugs carry side effects known or unknown, even after all the rigorous requirements of the licensing procedures which were discussed in Chapter 2. Medicines are administered to relieve symptoms, prevent ill health and in some cases provide a cure for illness. In some cases patients do not use the prescribed drugs and this non-adherence not only has a financial cost but can also increase illness through the development of drug-resistant organisms (Griffith, 2006). Carter and Taylor (2005) suggest that non-adherence can lead to ill health and reduced life expectancy in the case of medicines designed to reduce blood pressure; if the patient does not take the medicines, they are putting themselves at risk of having a catastrophic cardiac event such as a myocardial infarction (a heart attack).

Nurses have a **fiduciary** responsibility to their patients, who have entrusted their care to them. You are therefore morally bound to care for and advise your patients, and not to take advantage of them. At some time in the future you may be called upon to act as a patient's **advocate**, especially where competing interests are involved. Advocacy involves speaking on behalf of the patient and requires nurses to question and use their knowledge to support arguments where they feel, for example, that medicine prescription or administration may not be appropriate.

The Essential Skills Clusters are designed to provide the nurse with skills needed to make reliable judgements while ensuring safe and effective practice. Medicines administration is stressful at any stage in a nursing career but particularly so for newly qualified staff because of the knowledge and skills to be gained for entry to the register. All nurses should practise in accordance with an ethical and legal framework which ensures the primacy of the patient's interest. The *Standards for medicines management* were changed from guidelines to standards because they are not only for guidance but must be adhered to. As a student nurse wishing to gain entry to the register you need to increase your skill in using these standards. The standards themselves cannot meet all eventualities. The aim of this chapter is therefore to help you learn to make ethical and moral decisions for yourself by working through a number of examples and activities.

Morality and ethics

First we will consider why having a knowledge of **ethics** is important for you as a student nurse and how this relates to medicines administration. If you have no knowledge of ethics, you cannot care and protect those to whom you have an obligation.

Historically, there have been a number of ethical scandals relating to medicines, two of which are outlined here. After reading each of the case studies reflect on what these two incidents have in common.

CASE STUDY

In Willowcreek School in the USA between 1963 and 1966, children with learning disabilities in a residential setting were injected with hepatitis A to see how effective gamma globulin was and how the disease progressed.

Again in the USA, starting in 1932, in Tuskegee, 400 African Americans were persuaded by a nurse called Eunice Rivers to forgo antibiotic therapy for the sexually transmitted disease syphilis, even though the treatment was already known to be effective. This was part of an experiment that lasted over 40 years (Schwartz et al., 2002).

Each of these two true stories concerns unethical behaviour, and in each case one wonders why it was allowed to continue for as long as it did. One of the simple answers could be that nobody was prepared to question the activity that was taking place. People assumed that somebody else knew about it and that therefore it was all right. The question you have to ask yourself is, what should, could or would you do if you felt uncomfortable about how patient care or treatment is being delivered? To help you answer this question you need to understand ethics as well as having a consideration of the law as discussed in Chapter 2.

When relating ethics to medicines management a good starting point is to think about what can go wrong and why it creates an **ethical dilemma**. An ethical dilemma occurs in a situation where there are (at least) two options of how to act and:

- neither option appears to be satisfactory;
- there is a clash of values;
- the options themselves appear impossible.

Improving medication safety is the duty of all nurses. There is a **moral obligation** to disclose and report any errors.

Activity 3.1   *Decision-making*

Edwin Matthews is admitted to hospital in the middle of the night. Dr Liza McKenzie prescribes him a drug with which she is unfamiliar but which Mr Matthews assures her is the medicine he takes; in fact, he qualifies it with the statement 'I take two tablets every day.' Unquestioningly, Dr McKenzie prescribes the medicine. The nurse, Sally O'Brien, has to obtain the drug from an emergency cupboard and dispenses the drug to the patient who says 'These are different. I normally take the blue ones.' Sally considers this for a moment and suggests to Mr Matthews that they are probably just from a different manu-facturer, hence the different colour. Mr Matthews is given a medicine that is twice the normal prescribed strength and as a result of this he suffers an adverse reaction.

Activity 3.1 continued

First, think about how an incident such as this makes you, as a nurse, feel. Identify the issues that you think are right or wrong. Who was at fault – the doctor for the wrong prescription, the patient who gave the information in the first place, or the nurse who administered the medicine?

Discussion of this activity can be found at the end of the chapter.

As the nurse when it comes to medicines administration, you will often find yourself as the last person in a chain of events. This can create what is termed **moral distress**: the stress associated with ethical dilemmas. You may be faced with a problem that is not your fault, but is certainly your responsibility. Issues that can lead to moral distress in medicines management originate from problems caused by the professional relationships a nurse has with others. It may be a conflict over a drug prescription where you feel the dose is inappropriate or incorrect; it may be a lack of resources, for instance when an inferior type of wound dressing is prescribed because a more effective one is too costly. On top of that there are the everyday difficulties of just wondering what the right action to take is, when an alternative looks equally appealing. We call these decisions moral judgements and we make them based on moral values.

Values usually relate to things we consider important such as respect, fairness, freedom, dignity and happiness. There are individual values as well as societal values that help shape what we believe is the right or wrong course of action. Moral distress then occurs when the nurse holding a particular value finds that it is threatened in some way. Am I doing the right thing for my patient? Have I listened to my patient's reasons for refusing their medication? Am I ready to stand up and question my peers when I feel that the dosage they are prescribing or calculating is incorrect? At times we completely disregard the effect that such difficult situations might have on nurses themselves.

Patient safety in whatever setting is rightly regarded as an ethical imperative. Nurses have an ethical obligation to prevent and manage errors relating to medicines management. The NMC *Code*:

> requires all practitioners to conduct themselves and practise within an ethical framework based fundamentally upon respect for the well-being of patients and clients. While various rule-orientated and principle-based ethical models may assist in informing ethical decisions, within modern health care settings ethical dilemmas are by definition complex. Practitioners must recognise their moral obligations and the need to accept personal responsibility for their own ethical choices within specific situations based on their own professional judgement. In making such choices, practitioners must be aware of, and adhere to, legal as well as professional requirements.
>
> (NMC *Code*, 2008, p16)

Ethical theories

In order to consider the ethical issues in relation to medicines management, we first need to understand what ethics is and is not. The following activity gives you a chance to research for information.

'Ethics' comes from Greek and 'morals' from Latin; over the centuries they have come to mean more or less the same thing informally, but within a more formal setting such as

---

Activity 3.2   *Reflection*

What is the difference, if any, between ethics and morality? Using everyday terms with which you are familiar, describe such differences to a colleague.

Now try and think about what ethics is and is not, and write your ideas down in note form.

Discussion of this activity can be found at the end of the chapter.

---

healthcare, distinctions have been made. Morals can be seen as individual beliefs, whereas ethics is about the collective beliefs of a community.

Normative ethics is a branch of ethics that seeks to answer the difficult question of what 'norms' should help to guide us in the way we conduct our everyday lives. We are, of course, all individuals and as such we come with our own set of values, which can be described as beliefs or behaviour that we may share with others. Individual values originate from our customs or cultural background; they help to shape what we consider to be right and wrong, good and bad. They can allow us to undertake a certain action or disallow an action. Think back to being a child: who helped you to decide right from wrong, good from bad? **Bioethics** is a recent branch of ethics that is particularly concerned with ethical dilemmas that occur as a result of advances in biological sciences or medicine:

> The term 'morality' can be used either descriptively to refer to a code of conduct put forward by a society or some other group, such as a religion, or accepted by an individual, and 'ethics' is sometimes taken as referring to a more general guide to behavior that an individual adopts as his own guide to life, as long as it is a guide that one views as a proper guide for others.
>
> (Gert, 2004)

So in ethics we try to understand what is good or bad for individuals and society, but in order to promote what is good we need to identify factors that may impinge upon this.

Within an ethical framework we sometimes use the word 'rules' that can define our duties. Within nursing we have a professional role to undertake and we take on the moral obligations associated with nursing. Here you should revisit the NMC *Code* (2008) and try to identify what these obligations might be. Some are incorporated into professional behaviour, for example in terms of confidentiality or record keeping.

As nurses we have an ethical duty to support the health of our patients but this can cause an ethical dilemma. Let's look at another example in the following activity.

Activity 3.3   *Decision-making*

A patient with a cough goes to the Advanced Nurse Practitioner (ANP) because they feel they should have some antibiotics. The ANP refuses to prescribe them.

- What do you feel about this action? Is it right or wrong, good or bad?
- What could be the possible consequences for the patient?
- On what do you think the ANP based her decision?

Discussion of this activity can be found at the end of the chapter.

In order to understand how the nurse may have come to this decision we need to understand the different approaches to making an ethically sound decision.

Ethical frameworks can be described as a way of approaching ethical dilemmas while delivering care. Frameworks aim to help you in making decisions and you should familiarise yourself with those utilised in your own clinical setting.

In the next section there is a brief overview of some of the main ethical theories. Because of this brevity you should read further to develop your knowledge and skills. See the Further reading suggestions at the end of the chapter.

Teleological theories

Telos means end, and a **teleological theory** holds that the justification of an action is based on the 'ends' or consequences of the action. It is also referred to as **consequentialism**. This theory considers that the moral consequences of an action are the priority rather than the act itself. It is summed up as 'the ends justify the means'. The right course of action is the one with the intention of promoting the greatest good for the greatest number. **Utilitarianism** is teleological because it is the utility of the action that is important and the consequences for others are considered. **Egoism** is where the individual will undertake an action that will result in the best consequences for themselves; this action can be one that promotes happiness, pleasure or a sense of self-fulfilment. How does this translate to medicines administration? Consider the practice of national immunisation or vaccination programmes.

> ### Theory summary: the teleology of immunisation programmes
>
> The intention of national immunisation programmes is that society will benefit from not having to suffer the consequences of people contracting a certain illness, for example rubella (German measles). However, we know that no drug is completely safe and some people may be harmed as a consequence of immunisation. So how are such programmes ethically justified? A teleological approach might go something like this: contracting rubella can lead to life-lasting complications such as deafness; national immunisation for babies and young children from an early age can benefit society as there will be reduction in the number of people exposed to the disease. There will be fewer people requiring ongoing care throughout their lives and ultimately the disease may be eradicated.
>
> Nobody would dispute that we do not intend to cause harm to the baby or child by immunisation, and we seek to minimise the risk by carefully licensing drugs for human use, but we accept that there can be a minimal risk. So we go back to the premise of 'the greater good for the greater number'.

There are, however, problems with this theory. Suppose I intend to harm my colleague and I am successful; according to consequentialism I should be punished and many would agree that this is right. On the other hand, suppose I intend to help my friend and accidentally cause her harm; under the rules of consequentialism I should still be punished, because it is the outcome that matters.

For you as the nurse involved in such decisions the difficulty can be in identifying for whom an act is beneficial; if this is not possible, then the action ought to be the one that causes least harm.

CASE STUDY

The human papilloma virus (HPV) vaccine was developed in 2006 to prevent the infection that is now known to be a precursor to the development of cervical cancer and genital warts. Once the vaccine was made available by the pharmaceutical company Merck, there were a number of ethical dilemmas, which Lo (2006) outlined, and which are summarised below.

- Support for compulsory immunisation came from those who considered the consequences of the disease it was aiming to prevent.
- Opposition came from those who believe in abstinence from sexual intercourse before (and outside) marriage and believed that it would undermine social morality.
- Concerns within the media led to allegations being made that there were connections between immunisation and illness. In terms of the HPV vaccine they centred around development of thromboembolism and the neurodegenerative condition Guillain-Barré syndrome.
- Another form of opposition came from those who prefer to use complementary and alternative medicine.
- Other groups within society who believe in the right to self-determination did not like the government telling them what to do.
- Girls who opted out could be at a greater risk of developing cervical cancer in the future, but it could be argued that for all of us the future is unknown.
- Another ethical consideration was that it was unjust because it was offered only to girls and women within a certain age range.
- It was initially offered only to girls and women, who were considered to be the higher risk group, rather than boys.

So in terms of bioethics, what is the correct thing to do? The arguments presented here concern more than just science and religion: they relate to people being able to make **autonomous** choices.

The case study raises the issue of ethical dilemmas surrounding children and young people. We need to consider who should make decisions on behalf of children and young people and at what point in their lives they can make their own decisions. We refer to this as autonomy. Autonomy is the ability to make voluntary decisions about oneself based on adequate information that is provided without coercion. In relation to medicines management, it places a great deal of responsibility on you, as the nurse, to ensure that your patient is provided with this adequate information. In Chapter 2 we discussed the legal requirement of gaining the consent of your patient before any intervention; in the ethical domain this consent is seen to have two elements. The first relates to information-giving and the second is concerned with respecting patient autonomy.

When a patient asks you 'Are you sure I should be taking these tablets, nurse?' or says 'Tell me what I should do for the best', you need to answer appropriately so that the patient can then make their choice to take or refuse the medicines or other treatment.

Respecting autonomy in healthcare is also about changing the professional culture from a culture where 'Doctor knows best', which we refer to as medical **paternalism**, to an ethos of shared care, where patients are partners in their care.

Medical paternalism has no place in modern society; there should be a mutual respect for each other's skills, and your primary obligation should always be to your patient. As a nurse you will find yourself in a very privileged position of trust, and this should not be abused. You will develop knowledge about your patient's condition and disease process that they themselves may not be aware of.

Activity 3.4   *Communication*

Eric Jones is brought into the Accident and Emergency department where you are working. You are told that he may have suffered a myocardial infarction (heart attack).
   What information might you have that Mr Jones may not have?

Discussion of this activity can be found at the end of the chapter.

You should be mindful that any information you are given is not manipulated in such way that it could be misconstrued. For example, it would be coercion to steer a patient towards a particular choice, such as a less expensive pharmacological therapy rather than a more effective one. Even though you are studying adult nursing, you may come across children and those with learning difficulties or disabilities; these groups of patients might have a very different understanding of how medicines work in comparison to other patients, and we need to help them to express their anxieties and concerns for themselves.
   One area of ethical concern is when a nurse wishes to respect the patient's autonomy and therefore be beneficent, but disagrees or feels uncomfortable with the patient's wishes.

Scenario

Imagine you are working as a practice nurse in a primary care setting. Your clinic is involved in the human papilloma virus (HPV) immunisation programme. Mary Carter, a 22-year-old woman, says that after you have told her of the side effects as listed in the product information leaflet she now has no intention of being vaccinated.
   The next patient who comes for the immunisation is Jessica Blair who is 15 and comes to the clinic with her parents.
   Is there any ethical dilemma with either of these patients? How do we uphold the autonomy of all those involved in these two scenarios?

Here is a summary of the ethical issues surrounding these two clinic patients.

- If both Jessica and her parents agree to immunisation, there is no ethical dilemma.
- If Jessica and her parents were to refuse, it is acceptable so long as you as the nurse practitioner have given them adequate information to make that educated decision. This would also apply in the case of Mary. As a nurse, to use coercion to try to influence this decision would be unethical because it would be paternalistic.
- If Jessica asks for immunisation and her parents don't know, then this creates an ethical dilemma around whose interests should be met. Jessica's well-being and autonomy outweigh the right of the parent to make decisions on her behalf.

If we consider the options presented to us here, we can see how some originate from a consequentialist approach. However, this does not cover all the options, and a nurse could still be left wondering what the right course of action should be.

Deontology theory

This is a duty-based theory concerned with the rightness of an action rather than any consideration of possible benefit or harm as a result of the action. It is believed that the duty is self-evident, such as a duty not to lie and a duty to have respect for others. This theory tells you how you should care for others. There could, however, be some concerns with this theory for you as a nurse because it demands that nurses perform a duty regardless of the consequences. As a nurse administrating medicines, you are expected to consider any of the potential consequences such as the possibility of an adverse reaction. Another criticism is that it does not provide any guidance on what you should do where there is more than one duty and they clash.

Principlism

Tom Beauchamp and James Childress first published their book *Principles of Biomedical Ethics* in 1979. They described their work as somewhere between high level theory and common morality. The aim was to contemporise theories by proposing some ethical principles as a way of helping nurses make sound ethical decisions.

The crucial principles they identified were:

- respect for autonomy;
- beneficence (promoting benefit);
- non-maleficence (doing no harm);
- justice.

If we take each of these principles in turn, we will consider how they relate to medicines management in more detail.

Autonomy

Recently the world has been faced with an influenza pandemic. Should nurses be among the first to be immunised? You could argue they should, so that they can continue to care for their patients. This reflects a consequentialist viewpoint (the consequence justifies the act). However, how would you feel about compulsory immunisation? Would it be right to remove your autonomy in this way?

Now let's consider not you but those patients who face similar dilemmas when it comes to deciding whether or not to take their medicine or continue with a therapy regime, maybe because they are already suffering from the side effects of that therapy. If patients are concordant, then they are passive in their interactions – they do what they are told; it is a one-sided relationship in which their autonomy is not protected. If they are adherent, then they follow your recommendations but as a partnership. It is easy to see which kind of relationship you should promote in order to be an ethical practitioner. One way you can develop your skills is to listen carefully to the reasons your patient gives for not taking or questioning their medication.

Beneficence

Beneficence is a broad concept, roughly meaning 'doing good'; in ethical terms it encompasses any actions that bring about benefit or intentional good to others. Your patients will benefit if they are given accurate information, and society will benefit because the health of its citizens will improve. For you as the nurse, you can easily promote beneficence by acting as a facilitator. By facilitation we mean acting as an advocate for your patient, helping them to voice their concerns to other healthcare professionals. Consider the following scenario about a patient who suffers with Parkinson's disease. Parkinson's disease is characterised by a fine tremor usually in the hands, bradykinesia, slowness of movement, and rigidity of limbs as a direct effect of a reduction in the number of nerve cells that produce the neurotransmitter dopamine. Treatment regimes consist of specific drugs that either replace or mimic the actions of dopamine. The drugs must be taken at specific times of the day and because of the complexity of the therapeutic range it may take months or years to get the patient on the optimal treatment regime where there is a balance between their having smooth movement and no movement at all.

Scenario

Mrs Jacobs is admitted to your ward. The on-call doctor prescribes the drug levodopa for 10 a.m. and 10 p.m. You are on the night shift and when you come to give the patient her medication she is in a distressed state, saying she normally takes it at 6 p.m. and that she is losing the movement in one of her arms. She says she told the day staff, who said they would get the doctor to come back but they didn't. This lady is now clearly experiencing bradykinesia.
What can you as the nurse do now?

Ethically, the issue here is that the patient could potentially be harmed by an extended hospital stay and a breakdown in the therapeutic relationship. In this case the nurse on night duty cannot change the circumstances because the error was created by some-one else, so she should seek to do the least harm by ensuring that prompt medical help is sought. This act would be considered beneficent. Beneficence can be endangered in a number of ways, one of which is by not reporting errors, because it will deny nurses the opportunity to learn from the mistakes of others. The National Institute for Health and Clinical Excellence (NICE) in 2006 published a national guideline in relation to medicines administration and Parkinson's disease. As Mrs Jacobs's nurse, you should have a working knowledge of this document and promote this among your colleagues.

Non-maleficence

Non-maleficence is about minimising harm. Iatrogenic harm can be described as medically induced harm. The word *iatros*, from the Greek, actually translates as 'brought forth by a healer' and as such can relate to any form of treatment across healthcare settings. Indiscriminate use of antibiotics can lead to antibiotic resistance, and over-prescribing drugs such as opiates can lead to addiction. One of the biggest ethical dilemmas involving the iatrogenic effect of drugs relates to the drug thalidomide, which was introduced as a case study in Chapter 2.

One thing we have to remember is that the patients themselves have a vested interest in their own safety, especially when they question what we are doing. Rather than dismiss their questions it would be more ethical to engage in and promote the discussion. Patients are not trying to be obstructive; in fact, they are trying to keep themselves and you as the administrator safe.

Activity 3.5   *Evidence-based practice and research*

Look again at the case study on thalidomide from Chapter 2 (pages 42–3). A BBC documentary in 2004 (BBC, 2004) referred to it as one of the biggest tragedies of modern times. Having read the case study, can you identify any ethical concerns that might have been voiced at the time?

Do you think the medicine should still be available for prescription?

Discussion of this activity can be found at the end of the chapter.

Doctrine of double effect

As you saw from Activity 3.5, sometimes a medicine will have more than one physiological effect. The dilemma here, for you as the nurse, is which outcome is the least harmful.

Consider this example: opiates are very effective analgesics for severe pain but have an unwanted side effect, respiratory depression. Your patient Mrs Goldstein has been diagnosed with terminal carcinoma of the bronchus (lung cancer) with secondary bony metastases. Giving Mrs Goldstein the opiates relieves her pain, which is beneficent, but at the same time her respiratory function is deteriorating and she is at risk of respiratory failure, so giving her the opiates could be considered maleficent.

So how should you proceed? What is the ethical thing to do? From a **deontological** standpoint the consequences of respiratory failure possibly leading to death could be overlooked, because you as the nurse aimed to be beneficent and not maleficent: it is the act itself that is right or wrong. Consequentialists, on the other hand, would consider the outcome of the action. Here we need to have an understanding of what Mrs Goldstein feels about this treatment and death itself. If the patient equates death to pain and suffering, then death in itself would be considered a good thing; some people may consider a quick death better than a slower one. For you as the nurse this is very much about intention, and this must always be to promote beneficence. From a legal point of view, bringing about the death of another person or even assisting them in doing so remains illegal, as discussed in Chapter 2.

Justice

The final principle is justice. The term justice can be defined in a number of ways. Retributive justice is the justice that society expects to be served to wrongdoers, as a way of protecting society's values, as we saw in Chapter 2. In relation to medicines administration, the more common form of justice that requires consideration by nurses is distributive justice. Ethical dilemmas surround a patient's right to access medicines. An example of such a dilemma relates to the expense of treating patients with rare or 'orphan', even 'ultra-orphan', diseases. These conditions have a prevalence in a population within the European Union (EU) of less than 5 per 10,000 and the annual treatment costs can range from £50,000 to £300,000 (NICE, 2006a). To help reduce such dilemmas, agencies such as NICE produce guidance based on evidence of both **clinical effectiveness** and cost-effectiveness.

> **Research summary**
>
> NICE was challenged on a number of occasions in 2006 in relation to its own guidelines on the treatment of dementia. Access the NICE website and read the ethical arguments put forward by both sides in the dispute, to gain a better understanding of the importance of the ethical principle of justice.

Another example of distributive justice occurred in 2008 when more money was made available to Primary Care Trusts (PCTs) as a response to the rising measles outbreaks of 2006/7. Justice in healthcare is an issue not only on a national scale but also on a global scale. The World Health Organization, established in 1948, seeks to reduce corruption in the pharmaceutical sector (WHO, 2009).

> **Activity 3.6**   *Reflection*
>
> The four principles, as advocated by Beauchamp and Childress (2009), are listed below in alphabetical order. Now you have read about them, rearrange them in order of personal preference and find a colleague to undertake the same activity. Compare your list with your colleague's.
>
> - autonomy;
> - beneficence;
> - justice;
> - non-maleficence.
>
> *Discussion of this activity can be found at the end of the chapter.*

For someone new to thinking about ethics, the four principles approach can serve as a useful tool and a starting point when considering what one should do in any given situation. Beauchamp and Childress themselves have said in their book that there is no hierarchy to the principles. If this is the case, then anyone, including your colleagues, may consider one of the principles to have priority over another and this in itself may lead to conflict. In terms of conflict or dilemma, as nurses we need to understand what we should or should not do in every situation and we look for rules to follow. In Chapter 2 we looked at some of the legal rules that shape our practice; the NMC guides you with regard to professional and ethical practice by including consideration of ethical rules.

Ethical rules

There are some acts that are always wrong, no matter what the circumstances or consequences. Rules about such acts guide us in our everyday life; they allow or forbid us to undertake particular actions. One of the big questions of bioethics is whether there is a set of such rules that should apply at all times in any society. The difficulty we might be faced with as nurses is what to do when conflicting rules apply to a particular action. Do you give your friend your truthful opinion about her new boyfriend, or hurt her feelings? In healthcare we look to either institutional or professional codes of conduct for our answers. Our primary concern is patient welfare, and sometimes one rule might be sacrificed for another. For example, a doctor might decide to withhold the truth from a patient if they believe that telling the truth might cause the patient more harm. If we think back to Beauchamp and Childress's principles, we can see how a set of rules might be identified from these, such as: do not harm someone; do not lie or deceive; ensure promises are kept; and have respect for privacy. They identify these as universal principles of moral character:

- **veracity** or truth telling;
- privacy;
- confidentiality;
- **fidelity** or trustworthiness.

Veracity

Veracity is not just about conveying accurate and comprehensive information but also about the way in which it is delivered. Within a therapeutic relationship veracity is also about respecting others and keeping promises. Sometimes we try to explain something to a patient in such a way that we do not distress or frighten them, and we might be tempted to 'dilute' the information we present. We know that all drugs carry side effects and that the patient may experience an adverse drug reaction: we cannot know what the outcome might be after medicines administration. It is the patient's decision to make, and for this they require truthful information.

Nurses and other healthcare professionals may at times find themselves in a quandary about what to do when a patient is prescribed medicines but they appear reluctant to take them or lack the capacity to understand what they are for. In such circumstances nurses have been known to hide a patient's medicines in their food, thinking that it is in the patient's best interests. Their argument would be that doing so helps maintain the patient's health status; others see it as an infringement of autonomy. There are also practical problems: medicines that come in tablet form will need to be crushed in order to be mixed with food or drink. Harm could be caused to the patient from this very food/drink–drug interaction. For example, ampicillin (an antibiotic) is ineffective when mixed with food because it is destroyed by gastric enzymes. So as a nurse, the best course of action in the first instance would be to ask for advice about how the medicine might be administered in a different form, as it may be that the patient simply does not like the taste of the tablets. You are also respecting the autonomy of the patient in giving them a choice.

Withholding the truth, in whatever form, is deception.

Privacy

Privacy is an issue with several elements, such as having control over what others know about you and limiting access to information about yourself. Before the development of therapeutic cannabinoids for patients with multiple sclerosis, many patients would admit to illegally consuming marijuana for symptom relief of spasticity of limbs and visual problems. Many patients considered this information to be private, which created a dilemma for nurses who knew the drug might affect the therapeutic effect of any prescribed medication, potentially leading to harm. The issue for a nurse is whether they could or should tell someone about this.

We often talk about confidentiality and privacy as one and the same, but there are differences that you should be aware of in order to ensure you practise ethically. A breach of confidentiality occurs when the organisation responsible for keeping the information confidential fails to do so, or the organisation actually discloses the information without the patient's consent. If you were to walk onto a ward where one of your friends was working and read a patient's notes, you would be invading the patient's privacy, but you might also see confidential information at the same time. This would, of course, be both unethical and unprofessional.

Confidentiality

The NMC expects its registrants to respect people's right to confidentiality, and to ensure that people are informed about how and why information is shared to other members of the multidisciplinary team (MDT). Confidentiality is also about preventing re-disclosure of the confidential information. A ward pharmacist would be considered an essential member of your ward MDT, but you should still take care to divulge only information that is directly relevant to the medicines management of a patient. You have to ask yourself: does the pharmacist need to know all about the patient's personal circumstances and in what cases could such information be relevant?

Fidelity and trustworthiness

In order for patients to trust us as nurses they have to believe that the information we give them is given with regard for their interests. So if a patient tells you that he is worried that he may be experiencing side effects from his medication, he will expect you to do something with that information, even though he might not understand what that might be. You have a moral obligation to act on that information, and contact the prescriber immediately, telling the patient what you intend to do. You then tell the patient what you have done. You are giving the patient factual information, which we term fidelity.

In terms of medicines administration, a common example of patients questioning trustworthiness is when they ask 'Is that the correct dose? Are you sure you have the right amount?' When carrying out medicines calculations, one way to reassure patients is to be prepared to show the patient your calculations or to have them checked by a second person. If you gain consent before administering medicines, this will allow you to demonstrate respect for your patients' autonomy: you are allowing them to make the choice between accepting and refusing to take that medicine. Patients often worry that if they do not comply with treatments then all care will be withdrawn, and you as the nurse should ensure that your patients understand that they will be cared for in a non-judgemental manner at all times.

C H A P T E R   S U M M A R Y

All the statements in the NMC *Code* lead nurses to have a moral obligation to create an ethical environment, one that aims to reduce harm. Even as a student nurse you can be instrumental in helping to create this environment in relation to medicines management by becoming more ethically sensitive. This can be achieved by developing your knowledge of ethical theory and principles as well as participating in decision making relating to medicines management. The chapter aims to help you on this journey with a discussion and application of some ethical theory and principles across a variety of clinical settings. If you engage in the promotion of a safe environment, your patients and your colleagues will feel respected, knowing they will be listened to. Any nurse can be a patient's advocate by getting involved in any development of policy or guidance to ensure that ethical behaviour is promoted at all organisational levels. Sometimes ethics seems to make things more complicated: people involved in the decision making seem to offer more suggestions than answers. For you as a student nurse this can help you to identify those role models who can give good reasoned arguments as well as offer you the opportunity to engage in this activity, which will lead to an understanding of your own value and beliefs.

Activities: brief outline answers

Activity 3.1: Decision-making (pages 65–6)

In this first activity we need to consider what errors were made and explore the consequences. First, there were errors of omission, the failure to do something you should, in this case the careful checking of the product to be dispensed. Second, the omission led to a double dosage being given, which caused the adverse reaction.

A complacent nurse might assume that the correct dose is given without challenging the concerns the patient expressed when he suggested that the colour of the medicine was different. As a nurse you should always allow your patients to express any concerns they have as this will often prompt you to check what you are doing.

In terms of who was at fault you can see where the dilemma lies. It could be argued that it is the prescriber, but what about the dispenser? In the first instance this would not necessarily be the nurse – it might be the pharmacist who put the tablets in the emergency cupboard or it could be argued it is whoever collected those tablets and brought them to the ward. Always act on any concerns expressed by your patient.

Activity 3.2: Reflection (page 67)

To distinguish between the way we use 'ethics' and the way we use 'morals', consider the role of a criminal defence lawyer. Personally, they may believe that crimes such as murder are immoral and punishable, but ethically we would expect the lawyer to have an obligation to defend their client even if they know the client may be guilty of the crime. We expect them to behave *ethically* towards their client. They have a *moral* obligation to serve. Morals can be seen as individual beliefs whereas ethics is about collective beliefs of a community. You could read the introductory chapter in *Nursing Ethics* by Thompson et al. (2001) for further explanation of the historical development of ethical theories.

Activity 3.3: Decision-making (page 67)

A number of people might consider the action of this nurse to be inappropriate. After all, she has a duty to care for her patient (as we discussed in Chapter 2) so why should the patient not have the antibiotics? On the other hand, the patient is demanding a clinical treatment that many feel they need but that they may not need, or that the NHS cannot supply in all cases because of financial limitations. There are a number of consequences to be considered here. Without the antibiotics, it could be argued, the patient would get worse and might well infect others such as family members. Conversely, the antibiotics might make the patient worse, especially if they are prescribed inappropriately, as the patient may develop resistance to the medicine. There is also the issue that the patient may have an adverse reaction to the medicine. In this example the nurse is working in a specialised role. The nurse will have undertaken extensive training to allow her to carry out a thorough assessment of the patient's condition, and she will, as part of her role, be aware of the NICE guidance on respiratory tract infections, which offers information about antibiotic use, which she would utilise in making her decision.

Activity 3.4: Communication (page 70)

As the nurse in this situation you are likely to have information about the investigations that will need to be undertaken to actually confirm the diagnosis, as well as some idea of the potential treatment options. As a registered nurse you may also be included in the discussion about prognosis and what information should be shared with the patient. This patient is acutely ill with a potentially life-limiting condition. It would be wrong of any of the healthcare practitioners not to share the information with the patient, but the counter-argument would be that to share that information may actually cause the patient more harm. Here you are again reminded that the primary obligation from an ethical point of view is to your patient.

Activity 3.5: Evidence-based practice and research (page 73)

The drug thalidomide has been used since the tragedy occurred, but with stricter regulations. More recently it has been suggested – in the same BBC documentary (BBC, 2004) – that this drug, which caused so much devastation to people's lives across the world, might offer a new treatment option for people suffering from myeloma, a type of blood cancer. From a teleological, consequentialist or principlist standpoint we would say that no one else should ever be offered this drug again. If you are a patient with myeloma, you may well be prepared to accept the risks in the hope that the benefit outweighs them. In ethical terms this is where an act might have both good and bad effects, known as the double effect (Schwartz et al., 2002).

Activity 3.6: Reflection (page 74)

What is interesting about undertaking this activity is that when you compare your results with those of your colleague they may differ, and you may find yourselves arguing about which should come first. If we think they are all important, why should any one be first in rank order? Raanon Gillon, a long-time advocate of the principlist approach, suggested that autonomy should be 'first among equals' in an article he wrote in 2003 when he was reflecting on Beauchamp and Childress's contribution to bioethics (Gillon, 2003). Having ranked the four principles according to your own preference, access the article by Gillon and see if you agree with his argument that autonomy should be 'first among equals'. Gillon has also written a useful textbook called *Philosophical Medical Ethics* (1986).

Knowledge review

Now that you have completed this chapter, how would you rate your knowledge of the following topics? Remember that the knowledge you have gained should be commensurate with the expectation of the NMC proficiencies.

	Good	Adequate	Poor
1. Your understanding of the terms 'ethics' and 'morals'			
2. Identification of moral dilemmas relating to medicines administration			
3. How utilising ethical theory may help in decision making			

Where you're not confident in your knowledge of a topic, what will you do next?

Further reading

In relation to Activity 3.2 both these textbooks would serve as a good starting point:

Beauchamp, TL and Childress, JF (2009) *Principles of biomedical ethics*, 6th edition. New York, Oxford: Oxford University Press.

Thompson, IE, Melia, KM and Boyd, KM (2001) *Nursing ethics*, 4th edition. Oxford: Churchill Livingstone.

Useful websites

www.ethox.org.uk Website of the Ethox Centre, which is a multidisciplinary bioethics research centre in the University of Oxford's Department of Public Health. Its website contains a number of ethical dilemmas – not just ones related to medicines administration – that you could work through to develop and widen your knowledge of application of ethical theory, which can be useful when considering ethical dilemmas.

www.nice.org.uk The National Institute for Health and Clinical Excellence website, which has more about the work of the citizens' council and some of the ethical decisions it has been involved in.

Chapter 4

Pharmacology

Liz Lawson and Dawn L Hennefer

Draft NMC Standards for Pre-registration Nursing Education

This chapter will address the following draft competencies:

Domain: Nursing practice and decision making

2. All nurses must listen, recognise and respond to an individual's physical, social and psychological needs. They must then plan, deliver and evaluate technically safe, competent, person-centred care that addresses all their daily activities, in partnership with people and their carers, families and other professionals.

2.1. **Adult nurses** must safely use invasive and non-invasive procedures, technological support and pharmacological management for medical and surgical nursing practice. They must take account of individual needs and preferences as well as any existing or long term health problems.

9. All nurses must use up-to-date knowledge to decide the best way to deliver safe, evidence-based care across all ages. This must include knowledge and understanding of the essential content as set out within the standards for education in R5.6.1.

Domain: Professional values

8. All nurses must be responsible and accountable for keeping their own knowledge and skills up to date through continuing professional development and life-long learning. They must use evaluation, supervision and appraisal to improve their performance and enhance the safety and quality of care and service delivery.

Domain: Leadership, management and team working

9. All nurses must work within local policy to assess and manage risk effectively, reporting risk and raising concerns while maintaining the rights, wellbeing, security and safety of everyone involved in the care process.

Draft Essential Skills Clusters

This chapter will address the following draft ESCs:

Cluster: Medicines management

36. People can trust the newly registered graduate nurse to ensure safe and effective practice in medicines management through comprehensive knowledge of medicines, their actions, risks and benefits.

Chapter aims

After reading this chapter, you will be able to:

•   identify the different disciplines within pharmacology;
•   define pharmacokinetics and explain the different processes involved;
•   define pharmacodynamics and explain the different drug categories involved;
•   relate the principles of pharmacokinetics and pharmacodynamics to some of the more commonly seen drugs in practice.

Introduction

Medicines administration is a common activity within nursing, practised in numerous care settings. It is therefore important that as a nurse you understand how drugs work in the body. All drugs have side effects, some more severe than others, and because all patients are individual, we as nurses can never anticipate what side effects a patient will experience. We need to be aware of the potential side effects of drugs so that we can make the relevant assessments of patients.

The complexity of medicines administration requires nurses to draw on their pharmacological knowledge to ensure that the drugs that are prescribed are appropriate for the patient, that they are correctly administered and that the patient is involved in their treatment options and receives the correct information.

The pharmacological knowledge you will need is of:

•   nomenclature (what drugs are called);
•   pharmacokinetics (how the body deals with the drug); and
•   pharmacodynamics (how the drug works in the body).

This chapter will look at these aspects individually, aiming to demystify the terminology used and simplify the underlying principles of pharmacology so that you can build on your nursing knowledge to maintain patient safety in relation to medicines management. We will then go on to define some of the disciplines within pharmacology, including pharmacotherapeutics, pharmacogenetics, pharmacoepidemiology, pharmacoeconomics and pharmacognosy. You will also need to supplement your knowledge by using other resources, for example the *British National Formulary*.

The following chapter – Chapter 5 – will focus on the activity of administering medicines; it is important to remember that knowledge of medicines and administration of medicines cannot be separated in practice and therefore both these chapters need to be read to complement each other and help integrate your knowledge.

Sources of drug information

Drug developments and drug information change very rapidly. It is important, in terms of *The Code* (NMC, 2008), for nurses to ensure that the information they provide to patients is accurate, which means it needs to be up to date. Manufacturers' drug leaflets can be very informative for patients; however, some patients may find the print too small. For drugs that are dispensed in the clinical area the manufacturers' drug information may not be available, and so you will need to use other sources of information. You can refer to the *British National Formulary* (*BNF*), which is produced jointly by the Royal Pharmaceutical Society and the British Medical Association, but you also need to know how to use this publication and refer to the most recent copy. Local Trust policies must also be used as a source of reference, especially if your clinical placements are not confined to one particular Hospital Trust.

Definitions

A drug is legally defined as:

> Any substance or combination of substances which may be used in or admini-
> stered to human beings either with a view to restoring, correcting or modifying
> physiological functions by exerting a pharmacological, immunological or
> metabolic action or in making a diagnosis.
>
> (EU Directive 2001/83, cited in MHRA, 2007)

The word **pharmacology** is derived from the Greek words *pharmakon* meaning 'drug' and *ology* meaning 'knowledge or study of' (Thomas and Young, 2008).

Put simply, **pharmacokinetics** looks at how the body affects a drug. It relates to the body's ability to absorb a drug, as a drug has to enter the body to be effective. It relates to the body's ability to then distribute the drug to the site of action, and also to the metabolic processes required to make the drug suitable for elimination once it has had its effect. If the drug is not eliminated, it would remain continuously active within the body, with unwanted consequences.

Pharmacodynamics is the effect that the drug has on the body – in other words, how the drug works to achieve the expected effect.

To sum up, pharmacokinetics is concerned with how the body affects the drug, and pharmacodynamics is concerned with how the drug affects the body, that is, its mechanism of action.

Now we can look at some of the disciplines within pharmacology. Pharmaco-therapeutics is the study of how drugs are used to provide a therapeutic effect, such as analgesia to relieve pain or antibiotics to treat bacterial infection.

Pharmacy is the preparation and dispensing of drugs, and draws on pharmacokinetics, pharmacodynamics and pharmacotherapeutics.

Pharmacogenetics studies the individual variation in response to a medication because everyone's genetic make-up is different.

Pharmacoepidemiology looks at the benefits versus the risks of a particular drug as it relates to the spread of disease within populations. For example, in the case of swine flu (H1N1 virus), which exceeded epidemic status in 2009 and became pandemic, the British government made the decision to introduce a mass immunisation programme aimed initially at those individuals who are at the extremes of the age continuum and those individuals who have underlying health conditions such as asthma. Before reaching that decision, several issues would have been considered: do the benefits of having the immunisation and the potential side effects of the vaccination outweigh the symptoms and possible consequences of contracting the H1N1 virus? Another consideration would be the cost of this immunisation programme versus the cost to the NHS of treating those with swine flu. This cost-versus-benefit decision comes into the domain of pharmacoeconomics.

The study of medicinal plants is pharmacognosy. Out of all the disciplines within pharmacology, pharmacognosy probably best represents the history of pharmacology because it is the oldest; it has its roots in the study of natural drugs and their origins. These will be explored next.

The origins of drugs

The use of plants for medicinal purposes by prehistoric people was not accidental, although there must have been an element of trial and error. Some strategy was used, merely by observing how animals and people distinguished between the more palatable plants and the toxic ones. For example, the death of a person after eating a leaf from the deadly nightshade plant would inform the observer of its poisonous qualities (De Pasquale, 1984).

The source of every medical practice has long been associated with ancient Greece. However, the discovery in 1862 of an ancient manuscript in Egypt written on papyrus and dated 1555 BC refers to times as early as 3300–2600 BC and is concerned with 'preparation of medicines for all parts of the human body' (De Pasquale, 1984, p2). The manuscript reports on natural cures identified long before the first Greek doctor. From this papyrus it is noted that the ancient Egyptians were familiar with senna, castor oil and poppy, which are drugs still used today.

In ancient times the more knowledge gained by individuals about herbs and other potions and their effects, the more power these individuals had. They were held in high esteem because the effects of these herbs and potions were often seen to be magical (Page et al., 2002). Throughout the ages the properties of medicinal plants have been uncovered and explored by many a pioneer establishing their place in history, some of which are now described.

Pioneers in pharmacology and pharmacognosy

460–437 BC: Hippocrates collected and identified a large number of medicinal plants and used narcotics such as opium and mandrake. Because of his discoveries he was known as 'the father of medicine'.

384–322 BC: Aristotle noted more than 500 medicinal plants and their importance.

AD 57: Dioscorides wrote an extensive treatise on the practice of pharmacology known in Latin as *De material medica*. This document compiled a list of 500 plants and remedies related to these plants (Page et al., 2002).

AD 131–200: Galen described the pharmaceutical formulation of many plant and animal drugs (Bendick, 2002).

1493–1541: Paracelsus wrote about the poisonous qualities of substances and the relationship between when a substance is therapeutic and when it becomes toxic. He notably wrote *What is there that is not poison, all things are poison and nothing (is) without poison. Solely the dose determines that a thing is not a poison* (Bisset, 1991, p72). This proclamation remains the foundation of pharmacological thinking.

Herbal medicine today

Recently, there appears to be a growing interest in herbal remedies, which is reflected in the number of herbal stores we now see in the high street. Such is the growth in demand for herbal remedies and other alternatives to orthodox medicine that in 2009 the Department of Health published a document entitled *Extending professional and occupational regulation* (DH, 2009). Highlighted in this document is the recommendation from the Health Professions Council that healthcare groups including herbal medicine practitioners and traditional Chinese medicine practitioners should be statutorily regulated in the interest of public protection from unqualified practitioners. The Medicines and Healthcare products Regulatory Agency (MHRA) produce information on herbal remedies advised by the Herbal Medicines Advisory Committee, particularly when there are increased reports on particular remedies, for example St John's Wort (*Hypericum perforatum*), which is highlighted in the scenario below.

St John's Wort, *Hypericum perforatum*, is known to help relieve symptoms of mild anxiety and low mood (MHRA, 2008a) by inhibiting serotonin, norepinephrine and dopamine synaptic uptake (Guzelcan et al., cited in Andreescu et al., 2008). The use of this herb has spanned many years in the European community and has been effective; however, it has also been identified as interacting with other medicinal products, such as oral contraceptives, digoxin and warfarin, to name a few (MHRA, 2008a).

In 2008 the MHRA granted Bioforce (UK) Ltd a Traditional Herbal Regulation Certificate for 'Hyperiforce St John's Wort' tablets for sale without prescription. The decision was based on the applicant's demonstration of data that spanned 30 years of traditional use of St John's Wort, which included safety data. The following scenario surrounds the use of St John's Wort.

Scenario

You are on placement on a general medical ward where you are asked to admit a 66-year-old lady who has been diagnosed with a respiratory tract infection. You note the lady is hypersensitive to penicillin and that the doctor who initially saw her has prescribed erythromycin, which at present you are awaiting from the pharmacy. During further discussions the patient discloses she has been 'feeling down' recently and has been taking St John's Wort, which was recommended to her by a neighbour. She also reveals she did not disclose this information to the doctor because she did not feel it was important, as 'it's only herbal and not a proper drug'.

Activity 4.1   Communication

This activity is related to the above scenario. In order to answer these questions you need to read the following document: MRHA (2008) *Hyperiforce St John's Wort tablets* available at: www.mhra.gov.uk/home/groups/pl-a/documents/website resources/con020730.pdf.

- Are there any possible interactions identified when taking St John's Wort with erythromycin?
- If so, what would be the consequence for the patient if they took erythromycin with St John's Wort?
- Describe how you would use this information.
- What will you discuss with your patient?

An outline answer is given at the end of the chapter.

In relation to the increasing use of herbal remedies the MHRA (2008b) has identified that the public make the assumption that because the product is natural it must be safe. This perception can prevent the user from disclosing its use to medical and nursing staff and therefore possibly resulting in an incorrect diagnosis, as the potential cause of the symptoms have not been properly identified.

To summarise, it is important that the nurse provides an opportunity for the patient on admission to discuss all the drugs they take, including prescribed, herbal and over-the-counter drugs. Tact and sensitivity may be needed on the subject of illicit drug use, but nevertheless it needs to be discussed to maintain patient safety. Safety aspects in relation to medicines management will be addressed in Chapter 5.

Nomenclature

Nomenclature in pharmacology refers to drug names and their identification. Individual drugs can be identified in three different ways.

When a drug is being developed, its chemical composition is identified by a chemical name. As you can see in Table 4.1, ipratropium bromide is a drug that is used in the treatment of lung diseases such as asthma or chronic obstructive pulmonary disease (COPD). Its chemical name accurately represents its molecular formula but would be impractical to use.

The second way in which a drug is identified is by a **generic name**, which may be linked to its chemical composition. This generic name is the most appropriate name to use when the drug is prescribed (Galbraith et al., 2007). The generic name (rather than the chemical name) is used in the *British National Formulary* (*BNF*).

The third name that can be used to identify a drug is a brand name, noted by its capital initial. This is developed when other companies are entitled to produce the same drug and use the brand name to compete in the pharmaceutical market. Often a branded drug is more expensive when compared to the generic drug, but in a few circumstances a particular brand will be prescribed, as the patient *must* receive that drug. So, as shown in Table 4.2, a drug can have more than one brand name but it will have only one generic name.

Table 4.1: Every licensed drug has three names

Chemical name	8-azoniabicyclo (3.2.1) octane 3-3 hydroxy-1-oxo-2-phenylpropoxy-8-methyl-8-1 methylethyl bromide
Generic name	ipratropium bromide
Brand name	Atrovent®

Table 4.2: Some drugs have several brand names

Chemical name	Isobutyl propanoic phenolic acid
Generic name	ibuprofen
Brand name	Nurofen®, Brufen®, Cuprofen®, Calprofen®

Once you have identified the drug correctly from the prescription, you will need further understanding of the route of administration chosen. You will also need to consider the processes that the drug will undergo while in the body.

The next section will explore these areas in more detail.

Pharmacokinetics

For drugs to be effective they first have to enter the body, and to be beneficial they have to be of the correct concentration and act at the appropriate site of action. The choice of route for administration will affect the speed of the drug's action, and the dose will affect the concentration delivered to the tissues.

In an ideal situation all drugs would be delivered to the site of action directly, and indeed many drugs do work in this way, such as drugs that are inhaled to treat airway disease or creams for eczema that are applied topically. However, a more common occurrence is that the area to be treated is a distance away from the site of action; for example, drugs that are administered orally may need to be distributed to the kidneys.

The body has a number of important protective features that stop the entry of foreign materials such as viruses and bacteria, but these same features can also restrict the entry of drugs. Drug companies invest a considerable amount of money on research to design drugs that can overcome these anatomical barriers and to find the most appropriate methods for administering drugs to achieve the best absorption into the body, which ensures that the right concentration of the drug reaches the desired site of action.

Intravenous drugs given directly into the venous blood supply do not require absorption and so do not encounter the same problems as those drugs administered via other routes. It is important that the prescribed route of administration is followed.

Once drugs have been absorbed by the body they travel around the body in the circulatory system until the drug finds the site to act on. This process is called **distribution**. Unfortunately, most drugs are not very specific in their area of action so not only do they act at the desired site but they will also act on other areas of the body. This is the underlying principle in the development of common adverse effects usually termed **side effects**. An example is the painkilling agent morphine, which is given to reduce the activity of **nociceptors** (pain nerves). Morphine not only works to suppress the activity of the pain nerves (desired effect) but it can also act on the large intestine, giving rise to constipation (side effect). This is why kaolin and morphine can be used for occasional diarrhoea (*BNF*, 2010).

Next, drugs pass through the liver where they undergo a process of **metabolism.** Although the liver is capable of different metabolic processes involving drugs, the commonest is where the drug is prepared for elimination from the body, which is termed **excretion**. Drugs are most commonly excreted from the body by the kidneys and less frequently in bile and breast milk, or from the lungs and skin. For the kidneys to be able to excrete the drugs, they have to be metabolised by the liver.

In general drugs can be administered either:

- enterally, utilising the **enteral route** which is the gastrointestinal tract; or
- parenterally, using a **parenteral route**, that is, using bodily systems other than the gastrointestinal tract.

Enteral administration

Enteral administration uses the gastrointestinal tract for drugs to enter the body and includes oral administration, administration via a feeding tube and rectal administration, which we will now look at in turn.

Oral administration

This mode of administration is the most commonly used route for administering medicines and is generally well accepted by adult patients; the obvious exceptions are those patients who are unconscious or are unable to tolerate oral fluids. Some medications can be given **sublingually** (under the tongue) – see Figure 4.1 – as this ensures that the drug enters the body quickly. Using this route means that the drug diffuses through the mucous membrane, providing a direct route to the circulation leading to the heart. This route is used for administering glyceryl trinitrate (GTN), which is commonly used in the treatment of cardiac-related chest pain experienced in angina. Using this sublingual route quickly relieves the angina.

An alternative to using the tongue for the administration of drugs in the mouth is to use the **buccal mucosa**, the membrane lining the cheeks inside the mouth, as shown in Figure 4.1. Drugs can be inserted against the cheek or the gum and left to dissolve; for example, midazolam is used in this way to treat in the community patients who experience seizures. However, this is currently an unlicensed use, and you will need to receive the appropriate training (NICE, 2004) to be able to administer the drug in this way. Drugs administered using this buccal route can be used to directly treat ulceration of the mouth membranes; alternatively, this route can be used if the drug needs to be dissolved in saliva before being swallowed. The buccal route of administration may not be the most suitable if the patient has a dry mouth, as this will increase the time taken for the drug to dissolve and so will reduce its efficiency.

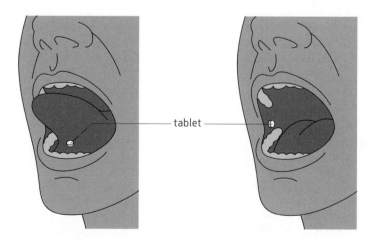

tablet

Figure 4.1: Sublingual and buccal administration

Drugs that are prescribed to be taken via the sublingual or buccal route should not be swallowed, as this negates the advantages of using this route; you will need to educate your patients about this.

Oral administration includes swallowing the drug into the gastrointestinal system. Drugs suitable for this route of administration are prepared as different formulations such as tablets, capsules, syrups and suspensions. This route of administration is common and has the benefit of being easy to conduct, convenient for patients to self-administer and painless. However, depending on the drug, the patient may experience an unpleasant taste. When administering a drug using the oral route, you should provide water to aid swallowing (McKenry and Salerno, 1998) as this will also help to protect the lining of the oesophagus from the effect of the medication.

Drugs taken using an oral route can have a direct effect on the lining of the stomach. This may be beneficial if this is the desired effect, such as when using an antacid, but the direct effect on the gastric lining may also be detrimental, such as when using aspirin. Medications administered using the oral route have to cross the villi walls in the small intestine to gain entry to the blood supply and to other body tissues. Although the oral route is commonly used, it is inappropriate if the patient needs to receive nil orally or has a vomiting illness, and may not be the most rapid method in an emergency situation.

The oral method of administration can also be inefficient, as not all of the drug may be absorbed by the villi of the intestine and some of the drug will be lost. The absorption of some medicines in the intestines can be influenced by the presence of certain foods and drinks, whereas other medications are not affected at all. This is because some medicines bind to the food molecules, reducing their ability to be transported through the villi, which will ultimately have a negative effect on the effectiveness of the drug treatment. For example, iron used in the treatment of anaemia should not be taken with tea or coffee, as both drinks reduce the absorption of iron, but instead should be taken with orange juice or cola as these fluids enhance the absorption. Some drugs carry precautions as they interact with certain foods. You will need to take this into account and check whether the drug you are administering will be affected by particular foods or fluids.

Scenario

You are in a medical speciality placement. A patient has a deep vein thrombosis and is being prescribed warfarin as an anticoagulant. You notice that the meal for the day is asparagus salad and the qualified nurse has noted on the patient's notes that they are not allowed this as asparagus and lettuce contain large quantities of Vitamin K.

Activity 4.2   Evidence-based practice and research

This activity is related to the scenario.

Look up this drug using the most recent *BNF* and answer the following questions.

- Why is the patient not allowed to have this meal?
- What effects on the action of warfarin do large quantities of asparagus or lettuce have?
- What would be the effect on the patient?
- Are there any fluids that can alter the effectiveness of warfarin?

An outline answer is given at the end of the chapter.

This activity has been included to make you aware of the importance of thinking about these issues in relation to drug absorption. Some other common drugs affected in this way include digoxin, used in heart disease treatment, which is not absorbed when taken with a high-fibre meal. The antibiotic erythromycin is destroyed by the high level of gastric acid produced when we eat, so this drug is better taken on an empty stomach.

Grapefruit juice contains a number of unique compounds that do not occur in other citrus fruit juices, and taking certain drugs with this drink may restrict their absorption. These include some of the drugs used to treat cancer, high blood pressure, heart disease and allergies, so you should ensure that your patients avoid swallowing grapefruit juice with their medications.

Alcohol should also be avoided when taking certain drugs because it can increase stomach acidity, which in turn exposes the drug to an increased amount of acidity, which may enhance the speed that the drug is broken down in the stomach.

It is therefore necessary to follow instructions related to oral administration and food or drink consumption and make sure that patients and carers are aware of them too.

The formulation of oral drugs is also relevant to when the drug is released and absorbed. Some drugs are termed **sustained release** as the way the drug is designed allows it to be released slowly and reduces the number of repeated doses needed. For example, a sustained release preparation of morphine can work for 12 hours, which will reduce the number of times the patient has to take this within each day.

Enteric-coated formulations such as the steroid tablets prednisolone EC have an outside covering that does not dissolve in stomach acid but does dissolve in the alkaline environment of the intestine. This provides the positive effect of protecting the lining of the stomach wall from the effects of the drug. As this enteric coating is important to the action of the drug, you should inform the patient that when taking the drug orally it should not be chewed or remain in the mouth for long as this provides an alkaline environment and the coating will dissolve in the mouth. A further instruction you should give for enteric-coated drugs is that they must not be given with alkaline-based antacids taken to treat indigestion, such as magnesium carbonate. This is because these alkaline preparations will dissolve the enteric coating in the stomach, which cancels the protective effect.

Scenario

Mr Smith has been admitted to the ward with worsening heart failure following a myocardial infarction seven years ago. In line with the NICE guidelines 2003 he is prescribed digoxin in addition to his regular medications. The nurse finds Mr. Smith has what he calls his 'indigestion tablets' with him, which she recognises as antacids bought from the supermarket.

Activity 4.3   *Evidence-based practice and research*

This activity is related to the above scenario.

Look up the drug digoxin in the interactions appendix of the most recent copy of the *BNF* and answer the following questions.

- What category of drug is digoxin?
- Why is finding out about Mr Smith's antacid tablets important ?
- Why should these two medications not be taken together?

An outline answer is given at the end of the chapter.

Feeding tubes

For patients who require nutritional support, feeding tubes may be sited either via the nose and into the stomach (nasogastric) or directly into the stomach (gastrostomy) or into the jejunum (jejunostomy). So when these patients require drug treatment, administration is usually via these feeding tubes. However, administration via this method requires special consideration because a number of drugs may interact with the feed being administered via these tubes. For example, drugs such as the antibiotic flucloxacillin or phenytoin, used in the management of epilepsy, should not be given when a nasogastric feed is in progress as these drugs will react with a milk feed, reducing the absorption by the intestine, and resulting in the patient receiving a lower dose than is required, which will lead to inadequate treatment.

When administering drugs in this way, you will need to involve and work closely with the pharmacist, who will make or provide a liquid preparation. For example, instead of paracetamol in tablet format you may want to request soluble paracetamol, which can be dissolved in water.

Crushing tablets followed by administration using a nasogastric tube may lead to blockage of the feeding device. The practice of crushing tablets may be a contradiction of the licensing agreement (see Chapter 2) and have potential negative effects on the patient. The pharmacist will provide you with a liquid formulation for administration via a nasogastric tube and will also calculate the amount of sorbitol being given to the patient. Sorbitol is a synthetic sweetening agent used in a number of 'sugar-free' formulations. A patient having too many 'sugar-free' formulations may develop diarrhoea, which would reduce absorption of the drug.

Rectal administration

This route can be used because the rectal mucosa, like the buccal mucosa, can absorb certain drugs, transferring them to the circulatory system. Rectal administration can be suitable for medications such as paracetamol when it is necessary to bypass the stomach, for example, in the case of a patient with severe vomiting or a patient who cannot take oral medication. The rectal route may be the route of choice to treat a local disease in the rectum, such as the insertion of steroids to manage inflammatory bowel disease.

One problem encountered by using this route is that of unpredictable absorption. The gastrointestinal tract has a variable blood supply, and absorption through the rectal wall is generally slower. Cultural differences may also influence the acceptability of this route.

Parenteral administration

Parenteral administration does not use the gastrointestinal tract and includes the intravenous, subcutaneous, intramuscular, topical or transdermal routes, and inhalation methods of administration, which we will now look at in turn.

Intravenous administration

Intravenous (literally 'within a vein') injections do not require absorption as they are administered directly into the blood supply. However, this route of administration can be hazardous for several reasons and you will therefore need specific training before you use it. This route of administration is useful in situations when either a prompt response is required or a high concentration of the drug in the bloodstream is needed at the beginning of a treatment regime. As a high concentration is achieved in the body quickly, any side effects can also be experienced quickly, so accuracy of dosing is vitally important.

The speed of action affects any allergic reactions, which will also occur swiftly. Allergic reactions can vary from mild to severe (anaphylaxis), such as experienced when using penicillin. You must be able to recognise the signs of an allergic reaction, seek prompt advice and act accordingly. This will be further explored in the next chapter.

Subcutaneous administration

A **subcutaneous** injection delivers a small **bolus** of a drug into the subcutaneous tissue of the skin. The subcutaneous tissue is located between the dermis of the skin and the muscle layer. The drug deposited into the subcutaneous layer will slowly diffuse into the blood supply of the skin. Because subcutaneous tissue has fewer nerves than muscular tissue, administration should be less painful than an intramuscular injection. This makes subcutaneous injections more suitable for self-administration than intramuscular ones.

Drugs can be administered into the subcutaneous layer by using syringe and needle, pen syringe devices, syringe drivers and infusions. Since the first subcutaneous injection 'pen' devices were introduced in 1985 to administer insulin there have been a number of significant technological advances in this type of injectable device (see Figure 4.2). Pen devices are available with a mechanism that gives an audible click when the dose has been successfully administered, which is particularly suitable for individuals with a visual impairment. Other pen devices have digital displays and memory functions displaying the date and dose of the last insulin administration. These pen devices can be disposable or refillable. You and your patient need to know how to dispose of these correctly to avoid a sharps injury, which will be explored in the next chapter. Whichever device is used you must ensure the correct needle length is chosen to ensure the delivery of the drug into the correct tissue.

A subcutaneous injection can be administered into the abdomen, the upper arms or the thigh. It is important for you to be aware that the speed of absorption of a drug into the circulation varies according to site. For example, an injection of insulin in the abdomen results in quicker absorption than an injection in the thigh, so the response to an abdominal subcutaneous injection of insulin occurs more rapidly than from one in the thigh.

You need to ensure that patients who need repeated subcutaneous injections change the site of administration frequently, as continual use of the same areas of skin can alter the structure of the fat tissue under the skin. **Lipoatrophy** can occur where the skin becomes hollow because some of the fat dissolves with repeated use of the same site. Alternatively, with repeated use of the same subcutaneous injection site the fat can

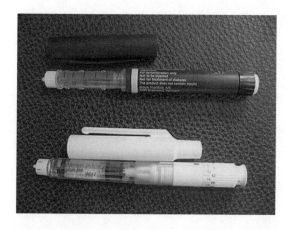

Figure 4.2: Insulin pens

increase, which is known as **lipohypertrophy**. This will give the skin a 'lumpy' appearance. It may be appealing to patients to use the same injection sites when they realise that using these areas can be less painful; however, you should advise the patient against reusing the same site as this prevents lipoatrophy and lipohypertrophy from occurring. Also, in the case of insulin therapy, using the same injection site can lead to unpredictable absorption of the insulin preparation, which can lead to erratic and unpredictable glucose control (King and Rubin, 2003).

Because of these skin-changing problems and the frequency of injections that patients with diabetes require, it is important that patients with diabetes have a skin examination every year, as recommended by Diabetes UK (2009).

Using the subcutaneous injection route is not a suitable choice when the patient is shocked or hypothermic as the physiological response to both of these conditions is for vasoconstriction of the blood vessels in the skin. This would lower the rate of absorption of the drug into the bloodstream and so reduce the therapeutic benefit.

Intramuscular administration

Unlike subcutaneous fatty tissue, muscle tissue is well supplied with blood and so some medications are administered using an intramuscular injection route when a more rapid response is required. Unfortunately, muscle tissue also has more nerve fibres, which can make intramuscular injection a more painful route of delivery.

You will need to select the correct site for administration into the muscle using anatomical landmarks. The site of choice for administering an intramuscular injection in adults is the **ventrogluteal** muscle. However, in children this is deemed to be an unreliable site for injection because of the difficulties in accurately placing the needle specifically at this site. The reason for this is the smaller muscle size of a child (Barron and Cocoman, 2008).

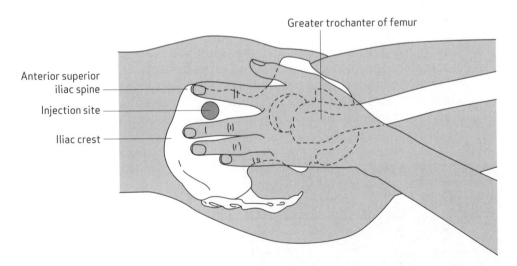

Figure 4.3: Ventrogluteal site for administration of intramuscular injections in adults

Topical or transdermal administration

A number of medications can be applied topically, meaning they are applied directly to the tissue requiring treatment. These include drugs used to treat the eyes, ears, vagina and the skin.

A number of drugs have now been developed that are applied transdermally (through the skin), often as 'patches', for systemic drug administration. When using patches the drug has to first penetrate the skin and then enter into the bloodstream. Drugs that can be delivered using this route include: glyceryl trinitrate (GTN), which is used in the management of angina; oestrodiol and progestogen, used in hormone replacement therapy; nicotine used as part of a smoking cessation programme; and fentanyl, used in the management of pain.

Patches usually contain a significant amount of the drug and people using them should handle them with care and wash their hands promptly after applying them. On the inner surface of the patch is a complex membrane that regulates the amount of drug delivered through the skin. It is your responsibility to ensure that your patient's skin is clean, dry and unbroken to gain the maximal adhesion and for the best effect. To help reduce the risk for potential skin reactions it is also advisable to regularly change the site of application.

One of the main advantages of transdermal administration is that the gastro-intestinal tract is avoided and so a constant concentration of drug delivery is achieved. These therapies are also well accepted by patients because they are non-invasive, painless and discreet. Also, treatment can be promptly and easily discontinued if it is no longer required or the medication needs alteration or changing to a different type, unlike an intravenous injection, for example.

The disadvantage of transdermal administration is that some patients may experience skin reactions, either because of the drug or the adhesive used to secure the patch to the skin. You need to be alert to these problems and take them into consideration when administering the drug via this method.

Inhalation

The lungs can be used as organs to deliver drugs such as anaesthetics into the body and can also be organs of drug excretion, which is the basis of the alcohol breathalyser test. The most frequent use of inhalation as the method for administering drugs is in treating the lungs and the airways directly for disorders such as asthma and chronic obstructive airways disease (COPD).

Use of an inhalation device provides local treatment directly to the site of the disorder, and the amount delivered to the rest of the body is minimised, which has the advantage of limiting the side effects experienced. You will need to help patients prescribed with inhalation medications to develop the correct technique of administration. An incorrect technique will deliver insufficient quantities of the drug to the precise area required; the patient will feel no benefit and their symptoms will persist.

There is now a vast array of different types of inhaler device available to choose from. When selecting a device with your patient, consider their age, manual dexterity, strength and preference as these may limit the suitability of some devices.

The routes of parenteral drug administration we have looked at are the more common routes, but you need to be aware of other less common but more specific parenteral methods used to administer drugs. These include intra-arterial, intra-articular, intradermal, intrathecal, intrapleural and intra-osseous.

Further information on these can be found in the *Royal Marsden Hospital Manual of Clinical Nursing Procedures* (Dougherty and Lister, 2008).

Factors affecting the effectiveness of drugs

A number of factors influence how effective drugs are. This chapter has already explored some of the more obvious reasons why an individual may not respond to drug therapy, such as drug–food interactions, and drug–drug interactions. Other factors are equally as important for you as a nurse to consider, but they are not always so clear. They include age, gender, genetics, liver disease and kidney disease, and these will be addressed next. Psychological factors are also an important consideration and will be discussed in Chapter 6 in more detail.

Age

With advancing technology and improved health there is an increasing proportion of individuals aged 60 years and over in the UK, and these people need particular consideration in terms of pharmacology. Over 50 per cent of all NHS prescriptions are dispensed to this age group (Milton et al., 2008).

This increased requirement for medication can reflect some of the physical alterations associated with advancing age. Older people are more likely to have multiple disorders that will require multiple drug therapies, some of which may interact with one another.

When older people receive drugs that could affect their balance or reduce their blood pressure, you need to think about lowering the risk of incurring fractures if they fall. With time, the liver reduces in size, which can increase the time taken to break a drug down ready for elimination. Consequently, in older people a drug can remain active for a longer period of time, so they are more likely to experience side effects such as toxicity. You should be mindful of the potential for toxicity and ensure patient assessment is conducted. There is also an age-related reduction in kidney function, so the time it takes for the kidneys to eliminate a drug is longer in the older person, which also results in this patient group being more susceptible to side effects.

Gender

Although it has been known for some time that there are differences in response to drugs based on gender, the mechanisms for this difference remain undetermined. Currently under examination are areas of difference such as hormones, genetics, metabolism and physical differences as well as susceptibility to certain diseases. Presently, the evidence on gender differences is anecdotal, based on male and female differences in the ability to metabolise alcohol, tranquillisers and aspirins. One reason for this could be that many pharmaceutical drug trials **recruit** more males than females. It may be that recruiting increased numbers of females into drug trials may develop this area of research.

Genetics

Genetics plays an important role in an individual's response to drug therapies. It would appear that many drug therapies are affected by a person's genetic make-up, including those therapies used for the treatment of depression, pain, migraine, high blood pressure and epilepsy. Spear et al. (2001) propose that the reason for the different response between individuals is related to differing genes within the liver, which leads to people having different concentrations of enzymes available for drug metabolism. Individuals with low concentrations of liver enzymes thus develop high concentrations of a drug and so experience more side effects, while other individuals with a high concentration of liver enzymes eliminate the drug more quickly and thus encounter limited relief of their symptoms.

Currently, there is no available test to determine who will respond most appropriately to a drug or who will experience more side effects, but it is predicted that this will be a future development.

Liver disease

Liver impairment in patients can lead to an array of complex alterations in pharmacokinetics. Liver disease can result in a reduction in liver cell number, reduced concentrations of enzymes for drug metabolism or an altered blood supply, which can reduce the oxygen delivery to the liver cells and reduce their ability to metabolise drugs. It is difficult to generalise how to manage drug therapy for individuals with liver disease as it is hard to compare patients with even the same type of liver disease since the altered mechanisms in drug breakdown could be different. All drugs given will have an altered metabolism in patients with liver disease and the alterations will become severe as the disease progresses. Collaboration between you and other nurses, doctors and pharmacists is imperative to ensure therapy is safe and effective for this group of patients.

Some drugs can also be the *cause* of liver disease, such as over-dosage of paracetamol. The following scenario will require you to look at the metabolism of paracetamol and the effects that over-dosage can have on your patient, particularly in relation to liver and renal function.

Scenario

Paracetamol is one of the most common drugs used in the UK.

According to the Paracetamol Information Centre (2010), each year in England and Wales approximately 130 deaths can be attributed to paracetamol overdose.

A newly qualified staff nurse, Tim is working in an Accident and Emergency department. He is awaiting the arrival of a patient who is suspected to have overdosed on paracetamol. The patient is male, 19 years of age and conscious. This is the only information available to Tim at this time.

Activity 4.4   *Team working*

Paracetamol overdose

This activity is related to the above scenario.

- What factors does Tim need to consider that will impact upon the treatment to be delivered?
- Why do these need careful consideration?

Research how the liver metabolises normal doses of paracetamol and then answer the following.

- What is the normal recommended dose of paracetamol to be administered to adults in any 24-hour period?
- Name the toxic by-product of paracetamol metabolism.
- What is the protein called that helps to detoxify this toxic by-product?
- How do you think the treatment relates to this protein?
- What are the consequences to the liver and kidneys if treatment is not initiated within 24 hours of paracetamol overdose?
- Which members of the multidisciplinary team would be involved in this scenario?

An outline answer is given at the end of the chapter.

The above scenario highlights the dangers of taking more than the recommended amounts of a drug by using an example of a drug that the public perceive to be particularly safe. This again reinforces the notion that it is the dose that can make a drug a poison, but it also indicates that newly qualified nurses should be well versed in knowledge of pharmacokinetics and pharmacodynamics so that their nursing care in relation to medicines management is evidence based and safe.

Renal disease

The kidneys are the main organs involved in the elimination of drugs. If the kidneys are impaired, then there is the potential for drugs to accumulate, and the patient is then at risk of experiencing side effects or more harmful effects of toxicity. To reduce the incidence of these effects a reduction in the frequency a drug is given may be prescribed as this will allow extra time for the drug to be excreted before the next dose is given. Alternatively, a reduction in the dose with the usual frequency may be prescribed.

A number of drugs can be injurious to the kidneys and these are described as **nephrotoxic**. The kidneys are particularly vulnerable as they have such an extensive blood supply. Also, the specific kidney tissue can be sensitive to certain drugs, including amphotericin, which is used to treat fungal infections, and the aminoglycoside antibiotics including gentamicin. To reduce the potential for kidney damage when using these drugs, you should correct any dehydration or electrolyte imbalances. This is because the kidney attempts to conserve many substances under these conditions, and if you do not correct the dehydration and electrolyte imbalances, the kidney will be exposed to a higher concentration of the harmful drug. Some drugs that are administered require regular blood monitoring of the drug levels to ensure the concentration of the drug is not rising excessively.

Some drugs excreted by the kidneys can cause an alteration in the colour of urine. You will need to alert your patients to this expected change in colour to allay potential anxiety. In particular, the drug rifampicin characteristically changes the urine to a red/orange colour, while drugs such as indometacin and amitriptyline can make the urine green in colour.

To summarise, you need to be aware of the pharmacokinetic processes of absorption, distribution, metabolism and excretion as these influence the dose of drug prescribed, the frequency of administration and drug interactions. Another consideration for you as the nurse are patient factors, for example co-existing diseases that may affect metabolism such as liver disease or renal disease that can affect drug excretion.

Pharmacodynamics

To recap, pharmacodynamics is concerned with the way that the drug affects the body, in other words how it acts. The purpose of this section is to provide an overview of the basic principles of pharmacodynamics. It is outside the scope of this book to provide a detailed account of all the drugs you will encounter while in practice, but you do need access to such information, so consult the Further reading and Useful websites sections at the end of this chapter.

Drugs can be classified in different ways depending on their mode of action. The different modes of action are listed below and will be looked at in turn.

- replacement drugs;
- enzyme inhibitors;
- ion channel inhibitors;

- neurotransmitter substances or inhibitors;
- others.

Replacement drugs

There are a number of diseases that result in the body becoming deficient in a particular substance, and the role of the therapeutic replacement drug is to address that deficiency. Examples of replacement medications include:

- dietary elements such as iron and folic acid to treat anaemia;
- vitamin and electrolyte supplements such as vitamin D and calcium;
- hormones.

Hormones are the most commonly replaced body deficiencies. Numerous hormones can be replaced, but insulin and thyroid hormones are commonly prescribed replacements. Insulin replacement hormone is required in individuals with Type 1 diabetes and can be given to patients with Type 2 diabetes when they continue to have poor blood glucose control despite using tablets and dietary alteration. Thyroid hormones are prescribed for patients who have an underactive thyroid gland and therefore a thyroid gland hormone deficiency. These hormones can be replaced in tablet form because they are not degraded by the stomach.

Enzyme inhibitors

An **enzyme** is a chemical catalyst that speeds up a chemical reaction. Enzymes are made of protein and usually carry the suffix '-ase'. A drug classed as an enzyme inhibitor attaches itself to a particular enzyme and stops its activity. This means that the chemical reaction cannot proceed (see Figure 4.4). An example of a drug that works by inhibiting enzymes is a statin, used to reduce blood cholesterol.

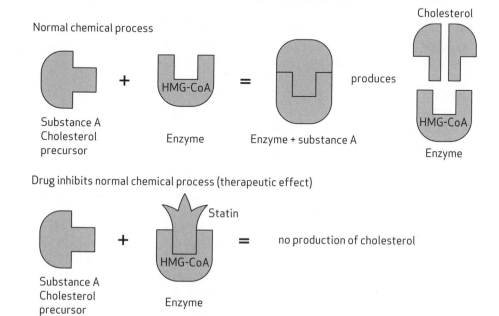

Figure 4.4: Action of enzyme inhibitors

Action of statins

In the liver there is an enzyme called Hydroxy Methyl Glutaryl-CoA reductase (abbreviated to HMG-CoA), which is involved in the production of cholesterol. **Statins** (for example, simvastatin or atorvastatin) are designed to recognise and bind to HMG-CoA enzymes. If the patient takes statins, then the drug will bind to the HMG-CoA reductase enzyme; this will make the enzyme inactive and the production of cholesterol will be markedly reduced, which achieves the desired effect.

Ion channel inhibitors

The movement of electrolyte ions in the body requires careful control otherwise they would move around the body randomly, which could lead to chaos and certainly disorganisation and dysfunction. To allow electrolytes into certain cells and tissues there are specific electrolyte channels. This means there are channels in muscles that are designed to allow only calcium to enter, which will then cause the muscle to contract. In nerve fibres there are channels that open to allow sodium to enter. When sodium enters a nerve cell an impulse signal is generated. Some drugs are designed to fit into an electrolyte channel to stop it opening. If the channel does not open, then a particular electrolyte is unable to enter and the function that usually accompanies the electrolyte entry will not occur. This is best illustrated by the following examples.

Calcium entry inhibition: calcium channel blockers for high blood pressure

When constriction of blood vessels is required, calcium channels open and allow calcium to pass into the muscle cells. When the calcium moves into the cell the muscles contract, resulting in a reduced blood vessel diameter; the blood is then moving through the vessel at a higher pressure.

In patients with high blood pressure, calcium channel blockers such as nifedipine can reduce the blood pressure. The drug will work by occupying the calcium channel and preventing the calcium from entering. This ensures the muscle does not contract but relaxes, causing a lowering of the pressure of blood inside the blood vessel.

Sodium entry inhibition: sodium channel blockers for dental surgery

For pain nerves to send the impulse of pain along nerve fibres, an influx of sodium into the nerve cell is required, which maintains the transmission of the pain signal. If a drug is given that is able to attach to the sodium channel and stop the entry of sodium, the pain signal will not be transmitted. An example is the lignocaine that is injected into the patient's gum at the dental surgery. Lignocaine occupies the sodium channels on the pain nerves, reducing the pain signal transmission while the dental work continues.

Neurotransmitter substances or inhibitors

One key feature of the nervous system is the anatomical gap called a synapse, the space between nerve fibres and muscles, glands and other nerve fibres. For a nerve impulse to traverse this gap, a **neurotransmitter** is released to activate the next nerve fibre in the sequence or stimulate the muscle or gland into the desired action. Refer to a standard anatomy and physiology text to refresh your knowledge on neurotransmitters.

Drugs can be used to act as false neurotransmitters; one such is salbutamol, which is used in acute asthma to signal to a constricted airway to dilate.

Drugs can also be used to *inhibit* a neurotransmitter from activating the next nerve fibre or tissue. For example, drugs such as ondansetron, granisetron and dolasetron are used to control vomiting by inhibiting the action of the neurotransmitter serotonin in the chemoreceptor trigger zone of the vomiting centre. Unfortunately, the large intestine uses the neurotransmitter serotonin for peristalsis so constipation is a commonly experienced side effect.

Other drugs

This final category is reserved for drugs that do not follow a mode of action comparable to the groupings we have already looked at. Their action is highly individual and includes drugs such as antibiotics, antiviral agents and drugs used in cancer therapy. Because these drugs do not follow the same pattern of action as outlined previously you should investigate the action of each individual agent.

The example given here is for the laxative agent called lactulose that is commonly used in the management of constipation.

Action of lactulose

Lactulose is a semi-synthetic sugar composed of fructose and galactose. Lactulose is taken orally, but this sugar is not digested as the gastrointestinal tract does not contain an enzyme called lactulase; it is not absorbed by the small intestine and does not enter the circulatory system. This undigested sugar is transported under the influence of peristalsis to the colon where the sugar attracts water into the colon. This increase in the water content of the faeces within the colon increases its bulk, which stimulates the colon wall and increases the water content of the stools, making evacuation easier (Chowdhury, 2006).

We have seen that pharmacodynamics relates to the mechanism of drug action, and we have looked at examples of replacement drugs, enzyme inhibitors, ion channel inhibitors, neurotransmitter substances or inhibitors and others. You will see examples of these drugs in your practice, and will need to read further about these categories so you can classify most of the drugs that you meet in practice, which will help you apply this pharmacological knowledge.

C H A P T E R   S U M M A R Y

Pharmacological knowledge is essential to the qualified nurse. The majority of patients in our care will at some stage of their treatment require pharmacological intervention, and the administration of this treatment will be the responsibility of the qualified nurse. We have a duty of care to our patients to keep them safe; this duty of care also includes any omission in care (NMC, 2008). We cannot administer drugs safely if we lack the fundamental principles of pharmacology, so what this chapter has outlined are the underlying principles, namely pharmacokinetics and pharmacodynamics.

Pharmacokinetics is concerned with how the body affects the drug; there are four essential processes involved in this, which in some way map the journey of the drug when administered. Absorption is the first process, which relates to the movement of the drug from the site of administration to the circulatory system. There are many routes involved in the administration of drugs, but the only route that avoids absorption is the intravenous route because the drug is directly injected into a vein. From the circulatory system the drug needs to travel to its site of action; this process is distribution. Before the drug can be excreted the process of metabolism occurs to change some drugs into suitable forms to be excreted. Although there are different ways in which the body excretes drugs, the main organ responsible for excretion is the kidney.

Because these processes are important in protecting the body you require know-ledge of the factors that can affect the effectiveness of drugs, for example, a patient's age and gender, and any coexisting diseases or drug therapies. This knowledge should complement your knowledge of drug action known as pharmacodynamics. In understanding the five categories illustrated, most of the commonly seen drugs within nursing practice can be placed within the relevant category. The inclusion of case studies, scenarios and various activities are designed to help integrate your knowledge with your practice and make it more memorable. However, you are advised to undertake further reading and study, using the sources provided at the end of this chapter. You are also advised to complement reading this chapter with reading the other publications mentioned at various junctures.

Activities: brief outline answers

Activity 4.1: Communication (pages 84–5)

There is a possible interaction between erythromycin and St John's Wort. If the patient takes erythromycin with St John's Wort, the consequence may be reduced blood levels of the drug erythromycin, which would result in a risk of therapeutic failure.

You should inform the nurse in charge, who should in turn inform the doctor who has prescribed the erythromycin, and also other qualified members of staff to ensure the drug is not administered while awaiting the prescribing doctor's arrival to review the patient. You should inform your patient that the information they provided is important and that the prescribing doctor also needs to be informed.

Activity 4.2: Evidence-based practice and research (page 88)

The high levels of Vitamin K in asparagus and lettuce will reduce the effectiveness of warfarin and increase the risk of further clotting. The patient's **INR** will be lowered and will need monitoring.

Fluids influencing the action of warfarin include cranberry juice, which increases anticoagulant activity, making the patient prone to excessive bleeding. Alcohol has a complex interaction with warfarin, itself acting as a mild anticoagulant. However, when combined with warfarin (dependent upon the alcohol drinking behaviour) it will adversely alter the management of the anticoagulation.

Activity 4.3: Evidence-based practice and research (page 89)

Digoxin belongs to the category of drugs known as cardiac glycosides. Finding out about Mr Smith's antacid tablets is important because it is necessary to know if patients are taking over-the-counter medicines that may interfere with the effectiveness of any prescribed treatments or drugs. Antacids should not be taken with digoxin as they reduce the amount of digoxin absorbed and the patient will not experience the expected benefits of digoxin. Mr Smith's heart failure will not improve and the symptoms will continue.

Activity 4.4: Team working (page 95)

The factors to consider are how many tablets the patient has taken, when they were taken (time period) and if they were taken with anything else, for example drugs or alcohol.

Knowing how many tablets the patient has taken is important, because if more than 12g in total or 150mg/kg body weight has been ingested and the patient has ingested them within the previous hour, activated charcoal should be administered. Activated charcoal can reduce the absorption of paracetamol into the gastrointestinal tract.

The administration of acetylcysteine (brand name Parvolex) offers protection for the liver if infused within 24 hours of taking the paracetamol. However, better results are seen if it is administered within eight hours of taking paracetamol.

The normal recommended dose of paracetamol to be administered to adults in any 24-hour period is 500mg to 1g in a single dose and not more than 4g in 24 hours.

The toxic by-product of paracetamol metabolism is *N-acetyl-p-benzoquinoneimine* (NAPQI).

The protein that helps to detoxify this toxic by-product is called glutathione. Acetylcysteine is a synthetic version of glutathione.

The consequences to the liver and kidneys if treatment is not initiated within 24 hours of paracetamol overdose can be fatal. As little as 10–15g (20–30 tablets) taken as a single dose or repeated doses within 24 hours may cause severe hepatocellular (liver cell) **necrosis**, although not as common renal tubular necrosis. In patients who have a higher risk of liver disease, for example those who are malnourished or are taking drugs that can induce liver enzymes, e.g. carbamazepine, St John's Wort and alcohol, may develop liver toxicity with doses as low as 5g in patients who weigh 70kg (*BNF*, 2010).

The members of the multidisciplinary team who would be involved in this scenario are paramedics, medical staff, biochemists, pharmacists and the mental health team.

Knowledge review

Now that you have completed this chapter, how would you rate your knowledge of the following topics?

	Good	Adequate	Poor
1. Definitions of disciplines related to drugs			
2. Nomenclature (naming system)			
3. Enteral routes of administration			
4. Parenteral routes of administration			
5. Factors affecting the effectiveness of drugs			
6. Five modes of action			

Where you're not confident in your knowledge of a topic, what will you do next?

Further reading

British National Formulary [59] (2010) London: BMJ Group and RPS Publishing. Available online at: www.bnf.org.
A very useful resource that provides expert information on medicine doses, side effects, contraindications and drug interactions.

Dougherty, L and Lister, S (2008) *Royal Marsden Hospital manual of clinical nursing procedures.* Oxford: Wiley Blackwell.
Provides details of numerous clinical skills based on available evidence.

NMC (Nursing and Midwifery Council) (2007) *Standards for medicines management.* London: NMC.
Current professional guidance provided by the regulatory body that sets the standards for many aspects of medicine management. The standards are devised to promote patient safety.

Useful websites

www.diabetes.org.uk The website of a charitable organisation providing authoritative information on all aspects of diabetes for professionals and the public.

www.mhra.gov.uk A useful site as MHRA is the regulatory agency responsible for ensuring that all medicines and medical devices are suitable for patient use.

www.nice.org.uk The website of NICE, an independent organisation providing guidance on a wide variety of illnesses and treatments.

Chapter 5

Medicines administration

Liz Lawson and Dawn L Hennefer

Draft NMC Standards for Pre-registration Nursing Education

This chapter will address the following draft competencies:

Domain: Professional values

8.   All nurses must be responsible and accountable for keeping their own knowledge and skills up-to-date through continuing professional development and life-long learning. They must use evaluation, supervision and appraisal to improve their performance and enhance the safety and quality of care and service delivery.

Domain: Nursing practice and decision making

2.1. **Adult nurses** must safely use invasive and non-invasive procedures, technological support and pharmacological management for medical and surgical nursing practice. They must take account of individual needs and preferences as well as any existing or long term health problems.

4.   All nurses must know the limitations and known hazards in the use of a range of technical nursing skills, activities, interventions, treatments, medical devices and equipment. This must include safe application and evaluation of the outcome in a variety of care settings, including complex, technical, diverse environments, to provide effective person centred care for people of all ages and backgrounds. Interventions will include safe medicines management, wound management, pain relief, and infection prevention and control. The nurse must report any concerns through appropriate channels and modify the plan of care to maintain safe practice.

Draft Essential Skills Clusters

This chapter will address the following draft ESCs:

Cluster: Medicines management

36. People can trust the newly registered graduate nurse to ensure safe and effective practice in medicines management through comprehensive knowledge of medicines, their actions, risks and benefits.

By entry to the register:

ii.   Applies knowledge of basic pharmacology, how medicines act and interact in the systems of the body, and their therapeutic action.
iii. Understands common routes and techniques of medicines administration including absorption, metabolism, adverse reactions and interactions.
iv.   Safely manages drug administration and monitors effects.
v.   Reports adverse incidents and near misses.
vi.   Safely manages anaphylaxis.

37. People can trust the newly registered graduate nurse to safely order, receive, store and dispose of medicines (including controlled drugs) in any setting.

By entry to the register:

ii.   Orders, receives, stores and disposes of medicines safely (including controlled drugs).

38. People can trust the newly registered graduate nurse to administer medicines safely and in a timely manner, including controlled drugs.

By entry to the register:

iv.   Safely and effectively administers and, where necessary, prepares medicines via routes and methods commonly used and maintains accurate records.
v.   Supervises and teaches others to do the same.
vi.   Understands the legal requirements.

42. People can trust the newly registered graduate nurse to demonstrate understanding and knowledge to supply and administer via a patient group directive.

By entry to the register:

ii.   **Through simulation and course work** demonstrates knowledge and application of the principles required for safe and effective supply and administration via a patient group directive including an understanding of role and accountability.
iii. **Through simulation and course work** demonstrates how to supply and administer via a patient group directive.

Chapter aims

After reading this chapter, you will be able to:

*   safely administer a medicine under supervision identifying the correct patient, correct medicine, correct dose, correct route and the correct time;
*   apply basic knowledge of pharmacology (see Chapter 4) to underpin your practice;
*   demonstrate an awareness of potential errors so these can be minimised.

Introduction

In the National Patient Safety Agency (NPSA, 2009b) document *Safety in doses* it was identified that the NPSA had received 100 medication incident reports where the medication had caused death and severe harm. These were reported via the National

Reporting and Learning System (NRLS), which is a service managed by the NPSA that aims to improve the safety of patients in the NHS by collecting the safety incident reports from the NHS providers and reporting their findings. The worrying feature of these incidents was that the most serious incidents were caused by medicines administration error (41 per cent). It is essential therefore that nurses charged with the responsibility of administering medicines adhere to the standards set out by the NMC to minimise risk.

Your role as a nursing student in the administration of medicines is very much a collaborative role that involves the patient, the registrant, the prescriber and the pharmacist, and possibly others. Standard 18 of the NMC medicines management standards (2007, p41) states that *students must never administer/supply medicinal products without direct supervision*; this also relates to student midwives. NMC Standard 8 in section 4 explicitly explains the process. It is important that you do not see this process in isolation but as a part of the overall principles related to medicines management, which include legislation, policy and guidance, pharmacological knowledge, ethical practice and, most importantly, numerical ability. The NMC sums up this important part of care delivery thus:

> *The administration of medicines is an important aspect of the professional practice of persons whose names are on the Council's register. It is not solely a mechanistic task to be performed in strict compliance with the written prescription of a medical practitioner (now independent/supplementary prescriber). It requires thought and the exercise of professional judgement . . .*
> (NMC, 2007, p6)

Standard 8 is guidance for the registrant, who has responsibility for helping you as the student nurse to achieve your competencies. In relation to medicines management, let us now look at the individual points within the Standard to see how they relate to you in your student nurse role.

Standards for practice of administration of medicines

The right patient
Standard 8 states:

> *As a registrant, in exercising your professional accountability in the best interests of your patients: You must be certain of the identity of the patient to whom the medicine is to be administered.*

It is essential to start as you mean to go on; if you establish good practice in every aspect of your care delivery and maintain your own personal standards, you will help to reduce risk. Whenever medicines administration is undertaken, it requires your full attention and concentration, which is sometimes difficult in busy clinical settings. Because of this, in some clinical areas staff wear, for example, a red tabard when medicine rounds are in progress, to signal to other staff members that there should be minimal interruptions when this aspect of care delivery is occurring. But whatever the system in place, it is the responsibility of the nurse administrating the medicines to ensure the relevant checks are carried out in accordance with policy to minimise harm to patients.

The process of administering medicines essentially starts with ensuring that the name on the **Patient Medicines Administration Chart** matches the identity of the patient for whom the medicine is prescribed. Safe patient identification is crucial in ensuring that the patient receives the correct care and helps to reduce errors.

In 2005 the National Patient Safety Agency (NPSA) produced a Safer Practice sheet that stated: *All hospital inpatients in acute settings should wear wristbands (also known as identity bands) with accurate details that correctly identify them and match them to their care.*

Patient identification

The wristband (identity band) should be placed on the dominant hand of the patient. It is usually completed following the admission process and generated at the patient's bedside, where possible, to ensure the correct wristband is applied to the correct patient's wrist. The rationale for applying the wristband on the dominant hand is that the non-dominant hand and arm tend to be used for administration of intravenous infusions or **venepuncture**, etc. so that the patient can maintain as much independence as possible (NPSA, 2005).

A wristband has a white background with black text, and the information on the band should be minimal; in 2008 another NPSA Safer Practice notice said that the national identifier should be the patient's NHS number and that this should appear on the wristband along with the patient's name and date of birth (NPSA, 2008). However, some healthcare providers stated they were unable to access NHS numbers, so this notice was reissued in 2009 with an amendment suggesting that the NHS number should be used when available, but that a hospital identifying number could be used in its place (NPSA, 2009a).

For those patients who cannot wear a wristband, for example because of a dermatological condition, or if a patient refuses to wear one or is unable to communicate (unconscious), then alternatives should be put in place (NPSA, 2005).

In some care settings, for example care homes where wristbands are not worn, photographs of the residents may be attached to their medicine prescription chart to identify individuals.

Final check

Before the actual administration of the medicine, there is a final check with the patient, either at the bedside or within the patient's home, etc. Where patients can communicate it is good practice to relay out loud the details on the patient medication administration chart and the patient's wristband so that the patient can spot any errors before taking the medicine.

Check for allergies

Standard 8 also states:

> You must check that the patient is not allergic to the medicine before administering it.

Another part of the checking process is to find out whether the patient has any allergies and/or hypersensitivities to particular medicines. These are usually highlighted on the Patient Medicines Administration Chart and, depending upon the severity of the allergy, may be documented on the front of the patient's medical notes. If the care provider has a wristband system for identifying allergies, then a red wristband should be used with black text on a white panel (NPSA, 2007). This system alerts the nurse immediately that the patient has an allergy, which then has to be identified.

Once the allergy has been identified, you require knowledge of the medicine prescribed to know if it contains anything to which the patient may be allergic. This information can be found in the *British National Formulary* (*BNF*) or the pharmaceutical company guidance. It is important that you do not assume the process of dispensing medicines is foolproof because other professionals can also fail to identify potential errors. The following scenario demonstrates this.

Scenario

A 36-year-old patient who was allergic to penicillin was administered Magnapen (co-fluampicil) intravenously. The allergy to penicillin was documented in the patient's medical notes, and the patient was also wearing a 'medical alert bracelet'. Following the administration the patient had a severe anaphylactic reaction that resulted in a cardiac arrest leaving the patient in a persistent coma (DH, 2004).

It is important to note that patients who are allergic to one penicillin will be allergic to all penicillins because the hypersensitivity is to the basic penicillin structure. Such people could potentially react to other **antibacterials,** for example cephalosporins (*BNF*, 2010). In the scenario above, the person administrating the medicine failed to recognise that Magnapen was the brand name for co-fluampicil, which contains flucloxacillin and ampicillin.

Here a number of questions are raised. Why was the generic name not used by the prescriber in the first place? Why was the generic name not identified when the medicine was dispensed from the pharmacy? Finally, why did the nurse not check to find out what the generic name was or refer back to the prescriber?

It is recommended that the generic or non-proprietary name be used when prescribing a medicine; however, the pharmacy may dispense a branded medicine. Normally, the pharmacist will identify that this is the same medicine, but this may not always be the case, so the nurse is required to look the medicine up in the *BNF*.

Patients in the community

Where medicines are administered in the community and in care homes the patient should be asked about any allergies; where the patient is unable to communicate effectively, the information should be documented where all staff can access it.

Whenever a medicine is administered you need to be aware that it may be the first time the patient has been exposed to the drug and so they will not know if they are allergic to it. The administrator should draw the patient's attention to the common side effects, and where the patient is not able to be monitored they should be encouraged to seek medical advice if they experience any side effects.

Knowledge of pharmacology

Standard 8 states:

> *You must know the therapeutic uses of the medicine to be administered, its normal dosage, side effects, precautions and contraindications.*

As we saw in the scenario, the system is not foolproof. Just because a medicine has been prescribed by a professional it does not mean mistakes cannot be made. If you are being supervised to administer a medicine, it is the responsibility of the registrant to ensure you know exactly what the medicine is and why the patient has been prescribed it. Some patients are well aware of the medicines they take regularly but may have had new medicines introduced into their treatment regime and so will need updating on the new medicines. There will be some patients who need clarification about the medicines they are taking and may need special instructions, for example whether to take the medicines on an empty stomach or after food (see Chapter 4). A sound pharmacology basis will prepare you for the different questions asked by patients and maintain patient confidence in the care they receive. Should you not know the therapeutic action of the medicine you need to admit this deficit in knowledge and rectify it before you approach the patient.

Activity 5.1   *Evidence-based practice and research*

What does the *Guidance on professional conduct for nursing and midwifery students* (NMC, 2009) say within 'Providing a high standard of practice and care at all times'?

An answer is given at the end of the chapter.

As well as knowing the therapeutic use of a medicine you need to be familiar with the normal dose range of medicines as well. Some drugs have a very narrow **therapeutic index**, which means that even a minimal deviation from the 'normal dose range' can be devastating to the patient.

The therapeutic index indicates the safety margin of a drug. If a drug has a wide therapeutic index then there can be large variations in the amount of drug a patient can receive before they experience side effects and the drug becomes toxic. A drug such as heparin has a narrow therapeutic index as increasing the dose can result in major bleeding.

If you do not know the normal dose of a medicine, then you will not recognise an abnormal dose, and the consequences of this to the patient could be harmful.

Before a drug is administered the nurse also has to consider precautions and contraindications. For example, if the patient is prescribed warfarin (an **anticoagulant**) you would need to consider any precautions associated with the drug that are clearly identified in the *BNF*. One such would be to check if the patient has bacterial endocarditis (inflammation of the inner lining of the heart, the endocardium). If warfarin is administered to a patient with bacterial endocarditis, it could increase the risk of bleeding (*BNF*, 2010).

In relation to contraindications, it is clearly identified that patients who have hypertension or have had a peptic ulcer should not be given warfarin. The nurse also has to think about other medicines the patient may be taking. For example, maybe the patient who is prescribed warfarin has diabetes and is taking tolbutamide. Here an awareness of pharmacokinetics is essential, because these two drugs compete for binding sites; warfarin can be displaced from its binding site by tolbutamide, meaning that the warfarin is free to act upon receptors and do the job it was designed to do. However, because of the amounts displaced it can cause haemorrhage. Other considerations are that some patients may have long-standing conditions, for example severe renal impairment, which contraindicate the taking of warfarin.

Care plan

You must be aware of the patient's plan of care (care plan/pathway).

The above discussion highlights the extreme importance of knowing your patient well in respect of their existing conditions as well as the condition being treated. If you are not familiar with the patient, then you need to inform yourself by reading the patient's care plan or notes.

Knowing the patient's details can alert you to recent decisions made about any changes to the treatment regime, which may include the need for the patient to receive nil orally until a procedure has been completed. The care plan should include past medical history, including liver and renal diseases, that would influence the choice of drug and the drug dosages prescribed. The evaluation within a care plan should indicate whether there has been any improvement in the patient's condition.

Is it the right medicine?

You must check that the prescription or the label on medicine dispensed is clearly written and unambiguous.

Unless the prescription is electronically generated, difficulties may occur in interpreting the handwriting. Any concerns about the prescription or about the information on the medicine box or bottle should be clarified before the medicine is administered and referred back to the prescriber. All the information on the Patient Medicines Administration Chart should be checked, starting with the patient details, then the medicine and dose, the start and stop date, prescriber's signature, time the medicine should be given and any instructions relating to the medicine. The stop date should always be noted; for example, a regime of antibiotics will be prescribed with a stop date so that the course runs over the correct number of days.

It is necessary also to look at the total dose that has been administered within a 24-hour period. For example, the recommended adult dose of paracetamol within a 24-hour period is 4g, which can be divided into four doses of 1g. However, by the time you come to administer the medicine the patient may have already had four doses of 1g. If the patient has taken the maximum dose but is still experiencing pain, the prescriber should be contacted and the patient reviewed.

The expiry date

You must check the expiry date (where it exists) of the medicine to be administered.

Before being administered all medicines should be checked for the manufacturer's expiry date, whether in a clinical setting or in a patient's home. Also check medicines brought into hospital by the patient, particularly if the patient has been assessed as capable of self-administration (see page 110).

Some medicines in the form of a suspension may need to be used within a certain time once opened, and so it is essential to document the date the medicine is opened. For example, eye drops when used in a hospital ward are normally discarded one week after opening, whereas eye drops being used in the patient's home can be used up to four weeks after first opening (*BNF*, 2010).

Any medicines that have expired should be returned to the pharmacy in accordance with local policy.

Other considerations

You must have considered the dosage, weight where appropriate, method of administration, route and timing.

You may need to calculate the actual dose of the medicine using a formula. Basic arithmetic and the formula(e) are discussed in Chapter 1. With certain drugs, and certain patients, it is essential to know the weight of the patient to identify the correct dosage required, for example when using anaesthetic drugs or with child patients.

Patient self-administration

Where patients are assessed as capable of self-administering medicines you should ensure that continued assessment takes place as appropriate and that records are maintained. Should any changes occur in the patient's condition that prevent self-administration, the arrangements for medicines administration should be altered to ensure patient safety (NMC, 2007).

Storage of medicines

For inpatients, the ward or unit may still have the traditional medicines trolley which is wheeled around to individual patients during the 'medicine round', although some areas now have locked cabinets attached to the bedside lockers. This locker system allows the storage of individual patient medicines, which may help to reduce errors. Care must be taken to empty their locker when a patient is discharged, as it is easy to overlook this and the next patient admitted is in danger of taking the wrong medicine.

All medicines must be stored in accordance with the manufacturer's guidance and in line with legislation and trust policy. Some medicines must be stored at certain temperatures and so are kept in a fridge. This will be a separate fridge from where food is stored and will not be situated in the kitchen but may be in a clinical room containing the controlled drugs cupboard. Schedule 2 drugs, which include opiates such as morphine and diamorphine, must be stored in a metal locked cupboard within a locked cupboard that is specifically designed to keep these drugs safe, in line with the Misuse of Drugs [Safe Custody] Regulations 1973. This cupboard should be situated where it is easily accessible to staff and can be observed. The way that the cupboard is also secured to a wall or floor is also specific so that the bolts holding it in place cannot be accessed from the outside. The key holder for these cupboards must be a qualified nurse or an authorised member of staff such as the pharmacist. There is also a requirement for regular auditing to maintain security and safety in relation to the storage of controlled drugs (NPC, 2009).

Preparation of the medicine

Once you have calculated the dose of medicine it requires preparing. In the case of a tablet it should be emptied into a clean medicine pot straight from the tablet bottle or blister pack, not being touched by your hands at all.

In the case of **suspensions,** the bottle requires shaking to mix the suspension as the wrong dose could be administered if not mixed first. When measuring the suspension into a medicine pot the lower **meniscus line** is the definitive line (see Figure 5.1). Syringes that are able to connect to an intravenous line should not be used when administering medicines, to reduce the risk of the medicine being administered via the intravenous route by mistake. Oral/enteral syringes should be used (NPSA, 2009b).

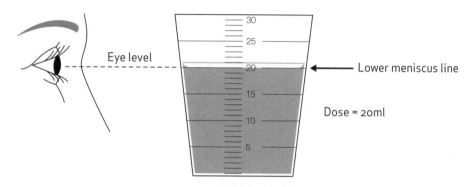

Figure 5.1: How to measure a liquid in a 30ml plastic pot

Controlled drugs

When you are preparing to administer controlled drugs (see page 110), more checks are required to ensure that each dose is accounted for. When controlled drugs are ordered by the qualified nurse they are ordered from a stock order book that has the signatures of those staff eligible to order them. When they arrive from pharmacy the nurse who receives them has a responsibility to enter them into the Controlled Drug Stock Book. Every time a patient is prescribed a controlled drug it requires an entry in the book to identify the date and time that the drug was administered, the name of the drug, the dose, the name of the patient, the signature of the nurse who administers the drug, the signature of the nurse who checks and observes the drug has been administered and a note of the remaining stock of the drug. It is also a requirement that all stocks of controlled drugs are checked regularly.

So what happens if the stock number of one particular drug does not match the actual amount?

Scenario

Mrs Wood has been prescribed 10mg of morphine to be administered intra-muscularly. Staff Nurse Hurst asks you to check and prepare the drug with her. You both go to the clinic and Staff Nurse Hurst unlocks the drugs cabinet and removes the **ampoules** of morphine. You open the Controlled Drugs Register on the morphine page and note from the stock balance that there should be 12 ampoules left. However, you both count only 11 ampoules. You ask Staff Nurse Hurst what you should do next and she suggests that you check through the previous entries. On doing so you see a mistake has been made: the previous entry stated that there were 12 ampoules of morphine left after the administration of 15mg of morphine. The morphine ampoules contain 10mg of morphine in 1ml of solution, and so 1½ ampoules of morphine where drawn up to make 15mg for the previous patient (5mg was wasted). But when you check the entry you note that although two ampoules were used, only one was deducted from the total and documented by mistake.

Most mistakes are genuine, and made for a variety of reasons, such as a momentary lapse in concentration or a distraction. The nurses who made the mistake should be informed so that they can clarify the error and learn from the mistake. Should, however, the case arise where there really is a missing controlled drug you should be aware of the procedure to follow within your area of work for reporting the incident.

You should also check that the formulation is correct; for example, if a sustained release morphine tablet is prescribed, a short-acting morphine tablet should not be administered by mistake.

Timing is critical for some drugs but sometimes not deemed important by the staff who administer the drugs. The NPSA in 2010 reported on the importance of timing and have called for action. They advise that for patients who are admitted into an organisation, the organisation should identify a list of critical medicines where the timing of their administration is crucial – medicines such as those used in Parkinson's disease, insulins and anticoagulants. Arrangements should be in place to advise staff of what to do when medicines are delayed or omitted. There should also be a review of the systems in place that manage the supply of critical medicines both in and out of pharmacy opening hours. The goal is to minimise omissions and delayed administration, and to highlight to staff that omissions and delays are patient safety incidents and should be reported (NPSA, 2010).

Knowledge of your patient

You must administer or withhold in the context of the patient's condition (e.g. digoxin not usually to be given if pulse below 60) and co-existing therapies e.g. physiotherapy.

Activity 5.2	Critical thinking

Why should you check the pulse of a patient before administering digoxin? Look up digoxin in the *BNF* to answer this question.

An answer is given at the end of the chapter.

Should you need to withhold medicines or omit them, for example, if a patient is vomiting and an alternative route cannot be utilised, this should be recorded on the Patient Medicines Administration Chart using the appropriate symbol. The patient should be reviewed to see if an anti-emetic can be prescribed and administered so that the required medicine can be administered as soon as possible. Alternatively, if a patient is taking nil by mouth you should speak with the prescriber before withholding their medicine.

Responsibility

You must contact the prescriber or another authorised prescriber without delay where contraindications to the prescribed medicine are discovered, where the patient develops a reaction to the medicine, or where assessment of the patient indicates that the medicine is no longer suitable (see Standard 25).

If you identify any contraindications you must contact the person who has prescribed the medication immediately so the medicine can be reviewed and changed. Before any medication is administered, the patient needs to give informed consent. This means the patient should be told about the benefits and common side effects of the drug, provided they have the capacity to understand the information. They can then make an informed choice as to whether they want to take the medicine or not. The common side effects of the drug are listed in the *BNF* and in the pharmaceutical company leaflet. You should tell the patient that if they experience any of the side effects, they should alert the nurse. However, it must be understood that it is your responsibility as the administrator of the drug to observe the patient regularly and complete the relevant assessments. For example, when captopril is administered for the first time, it is necessary to record the patient's blood pressure because a first dose can cause hypotension; it is advisable to start the medication at night and advise the patient to call for the nurse should they wish to get out of bed.

Record keeping

You must make a clear, accurate and immediate record of all medicine administered, intentionally withheld or refused by the patient, ensuring the signature is clear and legible; it is also your responsibility to ensure that a record is made when delegating the task of administering medicine.

Because you are a student nurse any information you record and any signatures you record on the Patient Medicines Administration Chart should be countersigned by the qualified nurse as they are accountable for any duties that they have delegated to you even if they are carried out under supervision.

Where medication is not given the reason for not doing so must be recorded.

When you have administered the medicine you need to record the date and time, dose and route on the Patient Medicines Administration Chart along with your signature and the registrant's.

You must be supervised at all times, as explained in Chapter 2, and your records should be clear and the handwriting legible.

Between September 2006 and June 2009, the NPSA received 21,383 reports of patient safety incidents that related to omitted or delayed medicines.

You may administer with a single signature any prescription only medicine (POM), general sales list (GSL) or pharmacy (P) medication.

Prescription only medicines can be administered with only a single signature from a registrant (NMC, 2007) although some policies dictate a double-checking procedure for prescription only drugs as well as controlled drugs, requiring two nurses to check medicines. You as a student nurse need to familiarise yourself with your organisation's policy and adhere to it. In all cases where you are being supervised you should always ensure you have a countersignature from the registrant who is supervising you.

Patient group directions

Patient group directions (PGDs) are specific written instructions for the supply or administration of a licensed named medicine including vaccines to specific groups of patients who may not be individually identified before presenting for treatment.

(NMC, 2007, p12)

Before a registrant can use a PGD they should be assessed as competent and identified in name within the document. In this instance the registrant must not delegate the administration of a medicine via a PGD and so you as the student are unable to administer under a PGD even if supervised.

Routes of administration

Now that we have looked at the process of medicines administration, let us move on to the different routes of administration and how you should administer via these routes using the processes outlined above. We will cover oral medications, injections, eye medicines, rectal administration, inhalations and oxygen therapy.

Oral medicines

Oral formulations include tablets, capsules and liquid solutions. This route can be used only if patients can swallow and have a functional gastrointestinal tract. The route is unsuitable for patients who are being given nil by mouth or who have a vomiting illness.

In conjunction with the NMC standards (2007), after washing your hands and selecting the medicine that corresponds to the prescribed medicine and formulation, the tablet or capsule should be placed directly in the medicine pot without touching your hands, either by opening the packaging of the tablets or by pouring the required number of tablets into the lid of the bottle, then transferring these to the medicine pot. If a scored tablet needs to be broken in half to provide the appropriate dose, local trust policy should be consulted and a tablet cutter should be used. The tablet cutter must be washed and dried after use. Disposal of the remaining half should be as per trust policy.

If the medicine is a solution, then prior to removing the cap and measuring the dose the mixture should be shaken well to ensure the contents are well mixed. Hold the bottle with the label in the palm of your hand as this will prevent the label from becoming unreadable should any medicine be spilled. If a liquid preparation is used, you must measure the medicine dose in a measuring pot to the lower meniscus for accuracy (see Figure 5.1). The top of the bottle should be cleaned prior to replacing the cap to prevent crusting of the neck of the bottle and the cap.

Oral medicines should ideally be taken with a glass of water to protect the oesophagus from the medicine and this should be offered to the patient if this is allowed. You must remember to follow any administration instructions provided about the timing of medication and intake of food, such as 'before meals' or 'with meals', as this may impact on the effectiveness of the medicine.

Oral medicines should not be left unattended on lockers or at the bedside in the hospital setting. The qualified nurse and the student should ensure that the patient has taken the medication prior to leaving the bedside as only then can the medicine be signed for and countersigned using the appropriate documentation.

If a patient is fed using a nasogastric tube or a gastrostomy device, then medicines administration using the gastrointestinal tract needs further consideration. Before administering drugs using these devices you need to be assured of the location of the device. Drugs can be administered using these feeding systems, but the pharmacist should be involved as they can provide a formulation suitable for administering this way. The pharmacist can prepare a solution based on the concentration of the medicine that will be suitably dilute so that the feeding device is not blocked.

If it is necessary to give a number of medicines to the patient using this route, then each medicine should be given separately and water flushed into the device between each individual drug. Using this method avoids the feeding tube becoming blocked and reduces the possibility of the two drugs reacting together in the tubing to form a clump that would block the feeding tube.

You will also need to take notice of any administration instructions that accompany the drugs from pharmacy prepared for use with feeding devices, as some medicines are not compatible with the liquid food being given. Some liquid feeds will interfere with the effectiveness of the medicine, inhibiting the medicine from being absorbed. The pharmacist will then provide instructions for the medicines to be given using the feeding device independently from the feed administration that must be followed.

Injections

Injections involve using a needle and a syringe. Injections can be given in a variety of sites including intradermal, subcutaneous, intramuscular, intravenous, intra-articular and intrathecal. Student nurses are usually involved in using the subcutaneous and intramuscular routes.

Before giving any injection you must follow the guidance in Standard 8 (NMC, 2007). Hand washing and the use of clean gloves are required for the administration of injections. You must ensure you provide privacy for this procedure as the skin will have to be exposed for the injection to take place. The practitioner and the student must take particular care to avoid needlestick injury, and the used needle must be disposed of into a designated sharps container using the local policy. Local reactions may occur at injection sites where the skin appears red, hot, swollen and painful, and this should be reported to the medical team for evaluation.

Subcutaneous injections

Subcutaneous injections are given into the fatty tissue that lies between the external layer of skin (the epidermis) and the muscle. There are a number of suitable bodily regions where subcutaneous injections can be inserted, including the abdomen, the lower part of the upper arm, the buttocks and the thigh. If patients need repeated sub-cutaneous injections, then the choice of site needs to be changed to prevent tissue damage to the skin. The needles used for these injections are shorter compared to intramuscular injection needles as the injection does not need to penetrate too far into the skin. Giving a subcutaneous injection usually involves inserting the needle at a 45-degree angle, but the shorter-length insulin injection needles should be inserted at a 90-degree angle.

Intramuscular injections

Intramuscular injections involve injecting the medicine into the muscle layer under the skin. There are five sites where intramuscular injections can be given:

- the deltoid muscle;
- the dorsogluteal muscle;
- the ventrogluteal muscle;
- the vastus lateralis muscle;
- the rectus femoris muscle.

An assessment of the patient's age, weight and muscle mass, and the amount to be injected, is required before selecting which would be the most appropriate muscle for injection. A different location would be chosen for an elderly patient compared to a younger healthy individual or, indeed, a child.

Ophthalmic medications

There are many different types of ophthalmic medicines that are prescribed for various eye conditions and for patients in various care settings. The medicines can be used diagnostically to gain an improved examination of the eye or therapeutically to treat eye injuries or conditions such as conjunctivitis.

Administering eye medications

A number of eye medications need to be stored in the refrigerator once they are opened. Any instructions on the label regarding storage should be followed. Unless the medicine preparation is for single use only, eye medications once opened should only be used for one week; however, if used in the patient's home, they can be used for up to four weeks (*BNF*, 2010). To prevent the risk of cross-infection or contamination, eye medications are reserved for a single patient and should not be shared between patients. If both eyes require treatment or examination, the label on the medicine should indicate which eye the preparation should be used for.

Procedure for instillation of eye drops

- Before commencing the procedure under the supervision of a registered nurse you must check the necessity for the administration of the eye drops and check this against the patient's details to determine if there are any known allergies.
- You need to gain the patient's consent to the administration of the eye drops and provide the patient with information relevant to the particular medicine. For example, you need to inform the patient of any potential alterations to vision, especially if the medicine is likely to cause blurred vision; in the case of a medicine with an anaesthetic action, the patient may have a reduced blinking reflex. The patient should also be told what to expect if the instillation is likely to produce sensations such as stinging or cold; you will need the patient's cooperation to instil the drops, and if they react to an unexpected sensation, it could be injurious.
- To administer the eye drops you will need to choose an appropriate area that provides good light, that maintains patient privacy and where the patient feels comfortable. After unlocking the refrigerator you must take particular care to remove the correct eye medication as many eye preparations are supplied in similar bottles. You will need to check with the qualified member of staff that the drug from the refrigerator matches the details on the prescription. Ensure that this is the correct drug and strength, that it has not expired and that it is clear which eye the medication has been prescribed for.
- You must then check the patient details against the prescription, again to check for any allergies and to confirm the correct identity of the recipient of the eye drops.
- It is essential that you wash your hands using a clinical hand-wash technique to prevent contamination.
- Before instillation of the eye drops it is essential that you assess the eyes to ensure they are clean, as any stickiness or exudates may interfere with the effectiveness of the treatment because the medicine will be unable to penetrate the debris.
- If the patient is capable, they should be instructed to lift the head upwards and backward to look towards the ceiling as this reduces the likelihood of the patient blinking and will aid the administration of the eye drops. The lower eyelid should be gently moved downwards; if the eye is swollen, then you must carefully manipulate the eyelid to reduce the possibility of further tissue damage. The bottle or dropper should be held in a vertical position and from a distance of 2.5cm away from the eye to be medicated to ensure the bottle or dropper does not touch the eye. The

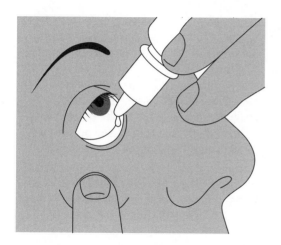

Figure 5.2: How to drop eye medication into the eye.

medication should be dropped into the lower fornix of the eye (lower lid) as shown in Figure 5.2.

- Following the administration of the eye medication, ask the patient to close the eye for approximately 1–2 minutes as this promotes the spread of the medication across the eye surface. Ask the patient not to squeeze their eyes tightly nor rub their eyes as the drops may be forced out of the eye unintentionally.
- Provide your patient with a clean tissue to wipe away any excess from their cheek.
- Return the eye drops to the refrigerator if instructed to, or if they are for single use then they need to be disposed of safely.
- Hand washing following the procedure is required again before continuing.

Once you have ensured the patient is comfortable, you must complete the necessary documentation, and as you are a student nurse this would be countersigned by the qualified nurse who has supervised you.

If there are a number of medications to be administered into the eye, it is preferable to wait 3–5 minutes before administering the subsequent eye drops as the eye can only absorb small volumes of fluid at any one time. Additional medication could be wasted as it will not remain within the eye for long enough. It is important that the patient is observed for the effects of the eye drops if this is appropriate; and you should monitor the patient for any potential side effects. Whether the patient is in an outpatients department or at home, they should be encouraged to look out for any possible side effects and inform the relevant professionals if they experience any. For those patients who have to travel, ask if they plan to drive: some eye medications used to examine the eye can dilate the pupils and distort vision, making it unsafe to drive.

Rectal administration of medicines

Medicines can be prescribed for administration via the rectal route for a number of reasons. This route can be chosen to treat a local disorder, for example in the treatment of inflammatory bowel disease or constipation. Using the rectal route enables medicines to avoid the upper gastrointestinal tract, which is preferable when a patient is experiencing nausea and vomiting, is to be nil by mouth or has a swallowing disorder. However, before you administer medicines via the rectal route a number of considerations need to be addressed.

- Initially, a risk assessment for moving and handling should be conducted, as ideally the patient needs to be positioned lying on the left lateral side with the knees flexed as this will allow the suppository or enema to follow the natural anatomical route of the rectum.
- Patient consent to this procedure is imperative, so you will have to provide information as to why the medication is necessary as well as why this is the preferable route of administration. You would need to explain to the patient what the expected effect of the medication will be and inform them of any potential side effects to ensure the patient can give informed consent in line with the NMC (2008) guidance.
- If this is the selected route for the administration of a drug, then essential to this procedure is the provision of privacy as this is an intimate procedure requiring sensitivity from the nurse to reduce patient embarrassment and maintain dignity (DH, 2003b).
- Again, you need to check the suitability of the prescription against the patient's details, then prepare the equipment prior to administration, which may include the moving and handling equipment (if necessary), disposable gloves, disposable apron, the prescription, the prescribed medication, lubricant, waterproof pad or bed protection, cleaning products, tissues and a clinical waste bag.
- In considering the area where the medication will be administered, you need to ensure that you can maintain privacy, that you can adjust the height of the bed, ensuring the brakes are securely applied, and that there are toileting facilities available as they may be needed quickly by the patient.
- Before starting the procedure you need to close the door or draw the curtains to maintain the patient's dignity. You need to verify the identity of the patient with the prescription. A waterproof protector should be situated under the buttocks of the patient but avoid unnecessary exposure of the patient by using clothing and bed linens thoughtfully. The patient may need assistance to adopt the correct position.
- You should now wash your hands and apply your apron and gloves.
- There is currently a debate about how a suppository should be inserted. It appears to be logical to insert the suppository using the shaped end first (Galbraith et al., 2007). However Abd-el-Maeboud et al. (1991) recommended that the blunt end should be inserted first. While this issue remains unresolved, the manufacturer's instructions should be followed. Prior to insertion the suppository should be lubricated. You need to separate the patient's buttocks and inspect the area for any visible bleeding. If this is found, then withhold the suppository until a medical review has been undertaken.
- Locate the anus and insert the suppository into the anal canal advancing approximately 5cm using the index finger and making a fist with the remaining fingers to avoid unnecessary contact with the genitalia.
- You can instruct the patient to take deep breaths if appropriate as this will help to relax the anal sphincter and reduce anxiety.
- On completion, wipe the area to remove any excess lubricant and assist the patient into an alternative position of their choosing.
- If the suppository is used for the relief of constipation, then it should be retained for the duration outlined within the manufacturer's guidelines.
- Dispose of the equipment used safely and wash your hands thoroughly. Complete the documentation, including the countersigning.
- Return to the patient to monitor for the effectiveness of the medication given and document any responses to the administration.

In relation to the administration of enemas the same principles should be used. The enema will usually be provided as a disposable package. The nozzle should be lubricated and the air should be expelled from the enema to minimise patient discomfort. The enema tube is inserted for 10–12cm to ensure the solution is delivered into the rectum, where it will be most effective, rather than the anal canal. Squeeze the enema fluid into the rectum, gently rolling the package up as you continue so the fluid does not flow backwards. The enema should be retained in the bowel for as long as specified in the manufacturer's instructions and again it is essential that the patient is informed of the location of the nearest toilet facilities (bedpan, commode or toilet) and assistance provided if necessary. Accurate documentation again is important to determine the effectiveness of the therapy.

Inhalation medications

Inhalation is a commonly used route of administration for medicines into the airways to prevent or treat diseases. Patients with asthma and chronic obstructive pulmonary disease (COPD) frequently use this method of drug delivery. Delivery of medicines in these situations can be prescribed in two forms: nebulisers and aerosol inhalers.

Nebulisers

Nebulisers get their name from the Latin for mist (nebula) as a nebuliser converts the medicine into a fine mist for the patient to inhale. A nebuliser is technically the chamber into which the medicine is placed. In the hospital setting the nebuliser can be connected to the compressed air or oxygen supply; in the community setting they may be connected to a mains- or battery-powered compressor. The mist of medicine created in the device needs to be inhaled into the airways so it is attached to a mask or a mouthpiece. Disposable nebulisers are available in the hospital setting, but in the community setting they can be washed after each use to avoid blockage and reused according to the manufacturer's instructions. The MHRA (2004) stresses the need to ensure reusable nebulisers are dried thoroughly as there is a recognised potential risk of transmitting infection, particularly Legionnaire's disease.

Aerosol inhalers

There are numerous hand-held aerosol devices available for the administration of medicines, particularly used by patients with asthma and chronic obstructive pulmonary disease (COPD). The advantage of this method of delivery is that the medicine is delivered to the site of action. These inhalers usually contain medicines for bronchodilation and steroids. Involving the patient in the choice of inhaler to be used is important as they need to be able to operate the inhaler to gain the most benefit. The drug within the inhaler is in a powdered form and the effectiveness of this type of treatment relies on the correct technique being used by the patient. The patients should be specifically trained by qualified nurses in inhaler technique, as poor symptom control is common due to inaccurate administration. Repeated assessment of the patient's technique is recommended. Spacers can be provided to enhance the accuracy of the patient's technique. A spacer is a plastic device with a mouthpiece at one end and to which the inhaler fits at the opposite end. The patient presses the inhaler to deliver one puff of the medicine into the spacer. The patient can then inhale the medicine through the mouthpiece. This can be repeated a number of times depending on the dose of medication prescribed. The spacer, like the nebuliser, must be washed and left to drip dry to prevent any medicine sticking to the side of the spacer device. The spacer should be replaced annually at least as recommended by Asthma UK (2010).

Procedure for administering an inhaler medication

- Under the supervision of a qualified nurse you need to review the prescription for the patient details and the drug prescribed.
- You need to ensure that the correct inhaler medication and device is selected for the individual patient from the locked cupboard.
- If the inhaler has a canister, you must check that this is firmly attached to the inhaler device. Then shake the inhaler to mix the medication within the canister and remove the cap from the mouthpiece.
- With the patient sitting upright, instruct the patient to exhale, then insert the inhaler into the mouth and close lips around it before inhaling.

Oxygen therapy

Oxygen as a form of therapy is only used on prescription, except in an emergency when it should be started immediately (BTS, 2008). Oxygen can be used either short-term or long-term and in hospital and community settings. Patients have individual requirements for supplemental oxygen, which is why it requires prescribing. Oxygen should be used with caution in patients diagnosed with COPD as a high concentration can be dangerous to the patient. Oxygen can be delivered via a face mask or nasal cannula depending on patient preference and the amount of oxygen prescribed. Nasal cannulas cannot deliver high concentrations of oxygen so when that is needed, an oxygen mask will have to be used.

Assessment of the patient is vital when they are receiving oxygen. You need to be able to assess the effectiveness of the oxygen therapy administered by using a thorough respiratory assessment. Being a gas, oxygen can easily dry the mouth and nostrils of the patient, so humidifying devices are used to reduce this effect. You should also ensure the patient receives sufficient fluid input throughout the treatment to prevent dehydration.

Because oxygen is a flammable gas, safety precautions must be followed when using oxygen therapy. No aerosols can be used in the vicinity of the oxygen: patients have experienced burn injuries from items such as antiperspirants and hairsprays used during oxygen therapy. Patients have also experienced facial burns as a result of smoking near an oxygen supply. In the home the same safety precautions apply to aerosols such as furniture polish and air fresheners.

Medicine errors

Whatever the route of administration used for a medicine, the nurse must always concentrate, giving care and consideration to the patient and all aspects of medicines administration. Most healthcare professionals strive to provide high standards of care but sometimes errors can occur; when those errors involve medicines the consequences can be fatal.

Between January 2005 and June 2006 the NRLS analysed about 60,000 medication incidents reported by NHS staff. The majority of these incidents (59.3 per cent) related to the administration process and involved one of the following:

- wrong dose;
- wrong strength;
- wrong frequency;
- wrong medicine;
- wrong patient;

- wrong formulation;
- wrong route.

In this final section of the chapter we examine some examples of such errors to demonstrate how they can occur and how to avoid them.

CASE STUDY

1. A prescribing error resulting in the wrong medicine being prescribed

Oxycontin (opioid analgesia) was prescribed in error; what should have been administered was oxybutynin, which is prescribed for urinary problems. Several doses were administered. The patient was also taking 15mg of MST (morphine-opioid analgesia) twice a day. So the patient was in effect being overdosed with opioid analgesics.

2. An administration error

Two staff nurses administered 2.5mg of oxycodone (opioid analgesia) via a subcutaneous injection. The patient was written up for 2.5mg Oxynorm (brand name of oxycodone) via the oral route only. The patient was already receiving oxycodone via a syringe driver.

3. A prescribing error that was not picked up when dispensed

A patient was administered 100mg/5ml of Oramorph (morphine), instead of 10mg/5ml. The prescription had been copied from the acute discharge note. However, the GP did not notice the error and the pharmacy also did not question the fact that the dose was ten times stronger than what had previously been dispensed. Fortunately, the patient noticed and so did not take the increased dose.

Activity 5.3   *Decision-making*

Errors such as those in the case studies occur far too frequently. If you notice a medicine error in the course of your work as a nurse, or by accident cause a medicine error, what should you do?

An answer is given at the end of the chapter.

Managing adverse events

If you observe a patient experiencing an adverse reaction to the medicine administered, you must inform the registrant. Remain with the patient so you can aid the registrant in any way to remedy the harm that may be caused by the reaction. The prescriber needs to be informed and all care documented in the patient's nursing notes. Once the patient is stable, the registrant can utilise the yellow card scheme, which is a reporting system that the Medicines and Healthcare products Regulatory Agency (MHRA) and Commission on Human Medicines jointly coordinate. Since 2005 patients have also been able to report adverse effects of medicines through this scheme.

Some adverse events can be avoided by meticulous practice to identify errors and therefore minimise risk. The final activities in this chapter will help you identify errors. All the Patient Medicines Administration Charts have been deliberately completed with errors, so look closely at each one and see if you can detect them.

Activity 5.4   *Critical thinking*

Farnsley Hospital Trust

Surname: BREVITT	Hospital ID: 979 2100817	Weight: 64 kg	Hypersensitivities —
First Name: MARJORIE	Ward: B23	Height:	
Date of Birth: 21 . 1 . 41	Consultant: GWJ		

Once only prescription

Date	Drug	Time	Route	Signature	Given Date	Time	Initials	Pharmacy

Regular prescriptions

Drug: CO - CODAMOL		Date	12/4/10	12·4·10	12·4·10	22/4/10			
Dose: TT	Route: PO	Time	06·05	10·10	14·30	18·35			
Signature:	Start Date: 12/4/10	Dose	TT	2	2	TT			
Pharmacy: DJ	Stop Date:	Sign	lw			TS			
Drug:		Date							
Dose:	Route:	Time							
Signature:	Start Date:	Dose							
Pharmacy:	Stop Date:	Sign							
Drug:		Date							
Dose:	Route:	Time							
Signature:	Start Date:	Dose							
Pharmacy:	Stop Date:	Sign							
Drug:		Date							
Dose:	Route:	Time							
Signature:	Start Date:	Dose							
Pharmacy:	Stop Date:	Sign							

You are working the night shift and are doing the medicine round with your mentor. Mrs Brevitt has requested analgesia. What would your actions be in answer to Mrs Brevitt's request?

An answer is given at the end of the chapter.

Farnsley Hospital Trust

Surname: HALLIWELL	Hospital ID: 127961	Weight: 75Kg	Hypersensitivities *PENICILLIN*
First Name: CHRISTOPHER	Ward: B9	Height:	
Date of Birth: 17/4/1955	Consultant: EAL		

Once only prescription

Date	Drug	Time	Route	Signature	Given			
					Date	Time	Initials	Pharmacy

Regular prescriptions		Time	Date 14/4/10	Date	Date	Date	Date	Date	Date
Drug: Tazocin		6.00							
Dose: 4.5g	Route: I/V	14.00							
Signature: NMJones	Start Date: 14/4/10	22.00							
Pharmacy: MA	Stop Date: 21/4/10								
Drug:									
Dose:	Route:								
Signature:	Start Date:								
Pharmacy:	Stop Date:								
Drug:									
Dose:	Route:								
Signature:	Start Date:								
Pharmacy:	Stop Date:								
Drug:									
Dose:	Route:								
Signature:	Start Date:								
Pharmacy:	Stop Date:								

Mr Halliwell requires intravenous antibiotics. You are observing the process. What do you notice about the prescription?

An answer is given at the end of the chapter.

Activity 5.6   *Critical thinking*

Farnsley Hospital Trust

Surname: Brendan	Hospital ID: 9473217012	Weight: 78 kg	Hypersensitivities NONE KNOWN
First Name: Willamina	Ward: B14 .	Height:	
Date of Birth: 30/4/39	Consultant: RI		

Once only prescription

Date	Drug	Time	Route	Signature	Given Date	Time	Initials	Pharmacy

Regular prescriptions		Time	Date 13/1/10	Date 14/1/10	Date 15/1/10	Date	Date	Date	Date
Drug: Atenolol		1000	FH						
Dose: 50mg	Route: PO								
Signature: Rivlin	Start Date: 13.1.10								
Pharmacy: 2L	Stop Date:								
Drug: Captopril		10.00	FH.						
Dose: 25mg	Route: PO								
Signature: Rivlin	Start Date: 13.1.10								
Pharmacy: 2L	Stop Date:	22.00	Bra						
Drug: furseride		10.00	FH.						
Dose: 40mg	Route: PO								
Signature: Rivlin	Start Date: 13.1.10 .								
Pharmacy: 2L	Stop Date: 14.1.10								
Drug:									
Dose:	Route:								
Signature:	Start Date:								
Pharmacy:	Stop Date:								

You are working a morning shift and looking after Miss Brendan. It is 9.45 a.m. on 14 January 2010 and you need to identify which drugs should be given. Which of the three medicines have you selected as suitable for administration?

An answer is given at the end of the chapter.

Farnsley Hospital Trust

Surname: FRENCH	Hospital ID: 127810	Weight: 71Kg	Hypersensitivities: None.
First Name: SARAH	Ward: C4	Height:	
Date of Birth: 1 / 10 / 1985	Consultant: DMB.		

Once only prescription

Date	Drug	Time	Route	Signature	Given Date	Time	Initials	Pharmacy

Regular prescriptions	Time	Date	Date	Date	Date	Date	Date	Date
Drug: Ceftriaxone	10.00							
Dose: 1g Route: IM								
Signature: SAL Start Date: 14/4/10	22.00							
Pharmacy: Stop Date:								
Drug:								
Dose: Route:								
Signature: Start Date:								
Pharmacy: Stop Date:								
Drug:								
Dose: Route:								
Signature: Start Date:								
Pharmacy: Stop Date:								
Drug:								
Dose: Route:								
Signature: Start Date:								
Pharmacy: Stop Date:								

Miss French has been admitted for treatment of a respiratory tract infection. The medical case notes state that Miss French requires 750mg intravenous cefuroxime. The mentor has suggested that this would be a good opportunity for you to practise your drug calculations. What are the mistakes on this prescription chart?

An answer is given at the end of the chapter.

Farnsley Hospital Trust

Surname: DOUGHERTY	Hospital ID: 274166	Weight: 104 Kg	Hypersensitivities Eggs
First Name: JOE	Ward: W 4	Height:	
Date of Birth: 12/6/1948	Consultant: ETB.		

Once only prescription

Date	Drug	Time	Route	Signature	Given Date	Time	Initials	Pharmacy

Regular prescriptions			Time	Date	Date	Date	Date	Date	Date	Date
Drug: Tolbutamide			8.00							
Dose: 500mg	Route: O		13.00							
Signature: CSLaws	Start Date: 14/4/2010		18.00							
Pharmacy: ZHA	Stop Date:									
Drug: Ibuprofen			8.00							
Dose: 200mg	Route: O		14.00							
Signature: CSLaws	Start Date: 14/4/10		20.00							
Pharmacy:	Stop Date:									
Drug:										
Dose:	Route:									
Signature:	Start Date:									
Pharmacy:	Stop Date:									
Drug:										
Dose:	Route:									
Signature:	Start Date:									
Pharmacy:	Stop Date:									

Mr Dougherty has Type 2 diabetes mellitus and has been admitted to your ward. The doctor has just reviewed Mr Dougherty and has prescribed ibuprofen for his pain. Can you identify what is incorrect about this prescription chart?

An answer is given at the end of the chapter.

Farnsley Hospital Trust

Surname: JABIN	Hospital ID: 932170791 13	Weight: 75Kg.	Hypersensitivities NONE.
First Name: WILLIAM	Ward: B21.	Height:	
Date of Birth: 4/7/45	Consultant: D.W.L		

Once only prescription

Date	Drug	Time	Route	Signature	Given			
					Date	Time	Initials	Pharmacy

Regular prescriptions		Time	Date 11/4/10	Date 12/4/10	Date 13/4/10	Date	Date	Date	Date
Drug: PERINDOPRIL									
Dose: 4mg	Route: PO								
Signature:	Start Date: 11.4.10								
Pharmacy: tw	Stop Date:	22.00	Luv	BH					
Drug: SIMVASTATIN									
Dose: 40mg	Route: PO								
Signature:	Start Date: 11.4.10								
Pharmacy: tw	Stop Date:	22.00	Luv	BLT					
Drug: PARACETAMOL		06.00	Luv 1g	BLT 1g	SEL				
Dose: 500mg - 1g	Route: PO	10.00	TH 1g	CuR	SU				
Signature:	Start Date: 11/4/10	14.00	TH 1g	CuR	SEL				
Pharmacy: tw	Stop Date:	22.00	Luv 1g	BLT 1g					
Drug:									
Dose:	Route:								
Signature:	Start Date:								
Pharmacy:	Stop Date:								

You are working the night shift on 13 April and you are reviewing Mr Dabin's medicine requirements. What actions would you take based on this prescription?

An answer is given at the end of the chapter.

`C H A P T E R    S U M M A R Y`

The purpose of this chapter was to provide you the student with a systematic way of administering medicines by utilising the NMC *Standards for medicines management* as a backdrop. Each requirement within Standard 8 was explored with the aim of maximising the therapeutic benefits of pharmacological treatments while maintaining patient safety and professional expectations.

To complement the administration process the common routes of medicine were also explored, providing useful procedural information. The chapter concluded with an overview of medicine errors and the management of adverse events with activities included to enhance awareness of potential medicine administration errors.

Activities: brief outline answers

Activity 5.1: Evidence-based practice and research (page 108)

Guidance on professional conduct for nursing and midwifery students (NMC, 2009) states, within *Providing a high standard of practice and care at all times*, that you need to recognise your limits of competence and work within your limits of that competence and always work under supervision. You also have a responsibility to ensure your skills and knowledge are up to date, that you always follow and adhere to employer policy and legislation and that the care you provide is based on best evidence. Finally, you should keep clear and accurate records.

Activity 5.2: Critical thinking (page 112)

Digoxin is a cardiac glycoside that works by increasing myocardial activity and reducing conductivity within the **AV** (atrioventricular) node (*BNF*, 2010), so it slows and strengthens the heartbeat causing the pulse to fall. If the pulse is already slowed to a normal range of 60 beats per minute, then the administration of digoxin will cause the pulse to reduce further with potential complications.

Activity 5.3: Decision-making (page 121)

You must first report the error as soon as it is discovered by informing the nurse in charge who will then inform the prescriber. You must ensure that the patient is also informed and assessed, monitored and treated accordingly. The details of your actions must be carefully recorded and steps taken to identify why the error was made so it can be prevented from occurring again.

The NMC views medicine errors more favourably when the nurse has made every attempt to keep the patient safe and has declared the error as soon as it was discovered.

Activity 5.4: Critical thinking (page 122)

When checking a prescription chart, the patient details and the drug information should be checked alongside when the last analgesia was administered. In the case of Mrs Brevitt, she last had some co-codamol at 18.35. However, if you check back through the day you note she has had three previous doses, which means she has had eight tablets in total. Although the dose of the individual tablets is not identified, the *BNF* entry for co-codamol shows the minimum amount of paracetamol in each tablet is 500mg and we know the maximum paracetamol that can be given in a 24-hr period is 4g, so Mrs Brevitt has had the maximum amount of tablets she can have in 24 hours. Because you cannot administer any more co-codamol and Mrs Brevitt is still in pain, you need to ask the prescriber for a different analgesic.

Activity 5.5: Critical thinking (page 123)

You should always work methodically through the prescription sheet so that you do not miss any mistakes. Therefore, check that the patient details match the patient, and look at any allergies. We note that Mr Halliwell is allergic to penicillin, so the next question should be whether the drug Tazocin contain penicillin. The *BNF* shows that Tazocin is the brand name for piperacillin and tazobactam. Piperacillin belongs to the penicillin group and so should not be given to Mr Halliwell. You should contact the prescriber.

Activity 5.6: Critical thinking (page 124)

In looking at the three drugs carefully you should have noticed that furosemide, the third drug on the prescription sheet, has been stopped. The stop date is 14 January 2010. The drug should therefore not be administered and to prevent any further risk the prescriber should cross out the drug so that staff can easily identify that it should no longer be administered. The remaining two drugs are correctly prescribed and so should be administered.

Activity 5.7: Critical thinking (page 125)

If we look at the prescription sheet we note that Miss French has no known hyper-sensitivities, so next we look at the drug. We know Miss French should be prescribed cefuroxime because it indicates this in her medical notes, but does the prescription read cefuroxime? It starts with 'Cef' as many of this type of antibiotic do, but the drug name is difficult to read. When we look at the dose prescribed it certainly is not the usual 750mg that should be prescribed. Because the dose is incorrect and the writing is illegible the prescriber should be contacted and the prescription card rewritten. The actual drug that has been prescribed is ceftriaxone, which is not the drug ordered for Miss French.

Activity 5.8: Critical thinking (page 126)

First look up the individual drugs in the *BNF* to check they are prescribed correctly. Also look at the prescription chart; note that the pharmacist has not seen the ibuprofen and has not signed the box to say it has been dispensed. The appendix in the *BNF* shows the interactions under antidiabetics, where you will see that NSAIDs can enhance the effects of tolbutamide, lowering blood glucose levels further. Ibuprofen should not be given in this instance and the prescriber should be notified.

Activity 5.9: Critical thinking (page 127)

Even though all three medicines have been administered for the last two nights, you should always check the prescription sheet carefully before you administer any drugs and not rely on the checks of staff who have previously administered the drugs. Start your checks by working from the top of the prescription sheet. The perindopril has been written correctly. The simvastatin, however, has not been signed off by the prescriber and therefore it should not have been administered. You can see that it has been administered for the last two nights and so you should inform the prescriber that the drug has been administered and ensure the prescription is amended. You should also ask your patient about their condition and if they have experienced any change. Your supervising mentor will need to follow the trust drug policy in relation to managing the drug error.

Knowledge review

Now that you have completed this chapter, how would you rate your knowledge of the following topics:

	Good	Adequate	Poor
1. The process for administering medicines			
2. The potential for medicine error and how to prevent it			
3. The process to be followed if an error is made			

Where you're not confident in your knowledge of a topic, what will you do next?

Further reading

Dougherty, L and Lister, S (2008) *Royal Marsden Hospital manual of clinical nursing procedures.* Oxford: Wiley Blackwell.
Provides details of numerous clinical skills based on available evidence.

NMC (Nursing and Midwifery Council) (2007) *Standards for medicines management.* London: NMC.
Current professional guidance provided by the regulatory body that sets the standards for many aspects of medicine management. The standards are devised to promote patient safety.

Useful websites

www.bnf.org The online *British National Formulary.*

Chapter 6

Partnership working

Liz Lawson and Dawn L Hennefer

Draft NMC Standards for Pre-registration Nursing Education

This chapter will address the following draft competencies:

Domain: Professional values

Adult nurses must also be able to promote the rights, choices and wishes of people of all ages in a wide variety of environments. They must work in partnership with a range of people with the aim of improving their outcomes.

5. All nurses must fully understand the different roles, responsibilities and functions of a nurse and adjust their role proactively to meet the changing needs of individuals, communities and populations.

Domain: Leadership, management and team working

Adult nurses must also be able to manage adult nursing care for individuals and groups, co-ordinate inter-professional care when needed, liaise with specialist teams and understand the role of other healthcare professionals. They must be adaptable and flexible and able to respond to the needs of people from all age groups and backgrounds. They must recognise the diversity of their role, particularly when working in environments such as accident and emergency, outpatient and walk-in clinics.

2.1. **Adult nurses** must manage the care of adults and young people across their healthcare journey recognising when to communicate with and refer to other professionals to deliver positive outcomes and a smooth effective transition between services and, where possible, to secure their preferred place of care.

8. All nurses must work effectively across professional and agency boundaries, respecting and making the most of the contributions made by others to achieve integrated person-centred care.

Draft Essential Skills Clusters

This chapter will address the following draft ESCs:

35. People can trust the newly registered graduate nurse to work as part of a team to offer holistic care and a range of treatment options of which medicines may form a part.

By entry to the register:

iii. Works confidently as part of the team and, where relevant, as leader of the team to develop treatment options and choices with the person receiving care and their carers.

iv. Questions, critically appraises, takes into account ethical considerations and the preferences of the person receiving care and uses evidence to support an argument in determining when medicines may or may not be an appropriate choice of treatment.

39. People can trust a newly registered graduate nurse to keep and maintain accurate records using information technology, where appropriate, within a multidisciplinary framework as a leader and as part of a team and in a variety of care settings including at home.

By entry to the register:

ii. Effectively keep records of medication administered and omitted, in a variety of care settings, including controlled drugs and ensures others do the same.

40. People can trust a newly registered graduate nurse to work in partnership with people receiving medical treatments and their carers.

By entry to the register:

ii. Works with people and carers to provide clear and accurate information.
iii. Gives clear instruction and explanation and checks the patient's or client's understanding relating to the use of medicines and treatment options.
iv. Assesses the person's ability to safely self-administer their medicines.
v. Assists people to make safe and informed choices about their medicines.

Chapter aims

After reading this chapter, you will be able to:

- consider the barriers to inter-professional practice and identify some strategies to overcome those barriers;
- demonstrate an awareness of the information required by patients so that they can make informed choices about taking their medicines;
- consider the reasons why some patients do not wish to take their prescribed medicines (non-adherence) and maintain their safety.

Introduction

Partnership working is essential in healthcare, and at the centre of the collaborative partnership is the patient. For if the patient is excluded from the partnership, then we have no business to be there. There are many terms used in the field of partnership working, for example inter-professional, multidisciplinary, multi-professional, inter-agency, all of which you will come across and need to understand. In this chapter we will be looking at partnership working within the context of medicines management. We will use the term inter-professional working to mean the working together of professionals (those healthcare workers who are professionally regulated) who have the common goal of ensuring that the patient's treatment, including pharmacological interventions, is effective and safe.

Before we discuss the different professions who have a responsibility in medicines management, it is worth reminding ourselves that healthcare has changed its emphasis from that of tending to the sick to one of preventative health promotion and education that endorses self-care and management. This is evident in the 'visions' listed in *Our health, our care, our say* (DH, 2006b), which include the following:

- people should be helped to remain healthy and independent;
- people should have choices and a louder voice to articulate their needs;
- service provision should increase in the home and community settings;
- services should be integrated and individualised;
- support for patients with long-term chronic conditions should be improved.

Within these visions, medicines play an important part, and the way that nurses manage medicines can influence a number of these directives. The NHS spends 10 per cent of its budget (approximately £10.6 billion) on medicines, and £100 million is the estimated cost of unused and unwanted medicines (RCGP, 2009), all of it paid for by UK taxpayers.

Over the last few decades there has been a political drive for nurses to work inter-professionally within health and social care. Several relevant documents have been issued by the government, including the Modernisation Agenda (Leathard, 2003). Many high-profile media cases have also concluded with recommendations for better partnership working and communication between professionals, agencies and other organisations.

Health professionals and potential barriers to medicines management

Despite the impetus to improve inter-professional working, in reality there are barriers that can sometimes affect the way in which we work together. This has been publically highlighted in the Shipman Inquiry, the Clothier Report and the more recent Laming Report. We will now examine some of these barriers.

All healthcare personnel have some responsibility for medicines management, whether they are professionals or not. Those who are directly involved have distinct roles in healthcare that we will discuss next; however, there are other healthcare workers who may not be directly involved but who have a responsibility to the individual patient and to the public to reduce risk and maintain safety.

Power differences

Traditionally, medical staff have had sole responsibility for prescribing medicines following medical assessments and diagnoses of patients' conditions. This tradition has been sustained for centuries and to a certain extent has facilitated the power imbalance that some healthcare professions feel exists between medical staff and other healthcare professions. This power imbalance is one of the potential barriers to professionals working together effectively. For you as a student nurse, working with medical staff can sometimes be daunting, particularly when working with more senior medical staff. Some student nurses may feel it is not their place to query the practices of other healthcare professionals; however, it is important to remember that we are all human and because of that fact unintentional mistakes are made. The key to effective inter-professional working is mutual respect, and the use of good communication and interpersonal skills that will provide you with the confidence to manage potentially awkward situations. What must be considered within your nursing practice is that patient safety is central, particularly where medicines are concerned. The consequences of errors can in some cases be fatal; tragedies hit the headlines every week. To explore this further, imagine yourself in the following scenario and identify the actions you would take, providing a rationale for your actions.

Activity 6.1   *Team working*

You are a student nurse in the first year of your nurse education. Doctor Ken Williams has asked you to prepare a trolley with the relevant equipment needed to insert a **peripheral cannula**, which he will be siting in Mrs Wood's hand. While you are preparing the trolley in the clinic room, you notice Dr Williams is drawing up some solution into a syringe but you do not know what this is. You take the prepared trolley to the bedside, and while Dr Williams explains the procedure to Mrs Wood you draw the curtains around the bed. Because you have been caring for Mrs Wood during the morning shift you remain with her throughout the procedure to assist Dr Williams and provide support for Mrs Wood. Dr Williams has completed inserting the cannula; with your help he has just secured it with a suitable dressing when his bleep starts to sound. He states he needs to leave and asks you to 'flush the cannula' with the syringe you saw him fill minutes earlier.

- What actions do you take?
- What could the consequences of your actions be?

In considering this activity you should familiarise yourself with standards 14, 18 and 20 of the *Standards for medicines management* (NMC, 2007).

An outline answer is given at the end of the chapter.

Barriers to communication

Communication is central in our everyday lives, both at work and in our social structures. There are many forms of communication, both verbal and non-verbal, and many skills are required to communicate effectively, especially in healthcare. How we communicate can affect all aspects of our work, and if we do not communicate well, this can hinder the care we deliver and the way in which we work with other professionals. Some examples of barriers to communication are:

- using jargon;
- poor record-keeping;
- illegible handwriting.

Terminology can be jargon; we are all aware of the increasing use of jargon used in today's society. In healthcare, different professionals use different terminology that can sometimes be alien to other professions, and certainly to service users. As nurses we are more sensitive to the use of medical and nursing terminology when communicating with our patients, families and carers, but do we consider this when communicating with a social worker or healthcare assistant? Using jargon or unfamiliar terminology can cause anxieties in those who do not understand it as well as causing frustration, making attempts at communication fruitless.

Written communication is also essential in healthcare, whether it be the Patient Medicine Administration Chart or the patient's notes. Care can be omitted, delayed or even delivered incorrectly when records are not kept, are incomplete or are not understood because of illegible handwriting or use of terminology that is alien to some professions. Overcoming these barriers can be simple if thought out. Electronic records may be helpful but not always available. Being careful with handwriting may take a little more time but is time well spent. If a medicine error occurs because you cannot read the prescription chart because the handwriting is illegible, the documentation you will need to complete will be extensive and time-consuming.

A lack of knowledge of other health professions

By the time you have completed your nurse education programme you should be suitably versed in what your nursing role entails. Guidance from the *Standards for pre-registration nursing education* (draft 2010) *The Code* (NMC, 2008), *Standards for medicines management* (NMC, 2007) and other policies and documents will inform you of your professional responsibilities and the boundaries of your practice that are in place to protect you.

We have identified earlier the traditional role of the medic, but what does the **pharmacist** do? Although pharmacists possess a sound knowledge of medicines and their management, their role has traditionally been concerned with the formulation and preparation of medicines, the preparation of feeds administered via nasogastric tubes, total parenteral nutrition and the dispensing of drugs, but not with prescribing. However, the advent of **non-medical prescribing** has changed that. Now pharmacists – and also nurses, physiotherapists, radiographers and optometrists – undertake non-medical prescribing.

Pharmacists and pharmacy technicians have a code of ethics comprising seven principles, one of which states:

> *pharmacists in the interest of their patients and the general public should use their professional judgement which may require health and social care professionals to be challenged if their decisions are deemed not to be in the best interests and safety of the patient.*

(RPSGB, 2007)

Their code also encourages partnership working with patients, carers and other healthcare professionals, maintaining respect for all. The principles of this code are very much in line with the code for nurses and midwives, which states that:

> *nurses should promote the health and wellbeing of patients, their families and carers and protect them by working with others. Within the managing of risk in this principle nurses and midwives are required to act without delay if they consider their patient to be at risk from a colleague or someone else.*

(NMC, 2008)

Are you, however, familiar with the roles of your colleagues in physiotherapy, occupational therapy and social work? Any lack of understanding of each other's roles between professions can widen the gap of a seamless service for patients. The best way for you to find out about the roles of other professionals is to ask them. Being a student commands supernumerary status, where your time is safeguarded for learning, so make good use of your opportunities to engage with other healthcare professionals now; in doing so you will start to build relationships.

Activity 6.2	Team working

The next time you get the opportunity, speak with the pharmacist about their role and responsibilities. Ask how you can work with them to ensure that patients receive the correct medicine on time and safely.

As this answer is based on your own research, there is no answer at the end of the chapter.

As nurses we have a direct responsibility for medicines administration, but as mentioned earlier within this chapter the advent of non-medical prescribing has now meant that registrants can engage more fully in the care they deliver making it truly **holistic** and providing it in a more timely manner.

Next we will discuss the emergence of nurse prescribing.

Nurse prescribing

For over ten years nurse prescribing has played an important part in care delivery. In 1999 a Department of Health report *Review of prescribing, supply and administration of medicines* recommended the recognition of two types of prescribers, an **independent prescriber** and a **dependent prescriber**. For patients with undiagnosed conditions the role of the independent prescriber is to assess and manage the care of the patient including prescribing. The dependant prescriber (now known as the **supplementary prescriber**) is responsible for managing the continuing care of patients who have initially been assessed by an independent prescriber and where prescribing may be part of the continuing care but will be limited.

In 2001/2 a succession of consultations took place between officials from the Department of Health and various professions on supplementary prescribers followed by further discussions with the Medicines Control Agency. These discussions were further considered at meetings of the Medicines Commission and the Committee on Safety of Medicines. After consideration by ministers, the Department of Health issued a press release in 2002 that exhibited plans that nurses and pharmacists should be developed as supplementary prescribers, enabling them to prescribe once a diagnosis had been made by a doctor (DH, 2003a).

This 2003 Department of Health guide *Supplementary prescribing by nurses and pharmacists within the NHS in England* provided information about supplementary prescribing (dependent prescribing), a rationale for advocating it, how it would work and who could undertake the role (DH, 2003a).

Since 2006 there have been further developments that allow nurses as well as pharmacists to extend their prescribing responsibilities. The rationale for this is that patient care will improve by enabling patients to receive their medicines more quickly, that the skills of healthcare professionals will be better utilised and that team working will become more adaptable. In nursing, the extension of prescribing responsibilities has allowed those nurses who prescribe from an extended formulary to prescribe any medicine to a patient with a medical condition, including some controlled drugs, as long as it is within the nurse's level of competence (DH, 2006c). Of course, these new powers are granted only once a nurse has successfully completed a recognised nurse prescribing course. This qualification must be recorded by the NMC before the role can be undertaken.

Indirect responsibility of non-professionals

There are numerous non-professionals who work as part of the team within hospitals and the community without whose services patient care would be severely affected. They include healthcare assistants, community care workers and hospital porters. Although in the majority of cases these individuals do not directly have a responsibility within the administration of medicines they may handle medicines in some way or be involved in the care of patients receiving medicines, so it is of vital importance that there is an awareness of the dangers of drugs and their omission. For example, the hospital domestic when cleaning around the bed area may notice medicines on the floor, or the community care worker may notice that the medicines in the dosette have not been self-administered by the patient they helped to dress that morning. Their responsibility would be to inform the registrant on the ward or the patient's GP to ensure that the patient does not come to harm by missing their medicines. The NPSA (2010) reported on the issues of patients not receiving their medicines (omitted), or not receiving them on time, and the impact this can have on patients' health. In 2006 The Parkinson's Society launched a campaign 'Get it on time', which highlighted the importance of individuals with Parkinson's disease receiving their medication on time to maintain their independence. Any untimely gaps in their treatment regimes can cause an increase in their symptoms and seriously affect their daily living activities.

Patients as partners in medicines management

Central to the effectiveness of medicines management is the patient's ability and willingness to take the treatment prescribed. Different studies indicate variable numbers of patients following a prescribed regime. Approximately 25–50 per cent of patients fail to follow the prescribed treatment correctly (WHO, 2003).

The latest report from the chief nurse for England, which provided a review of nursing careers, highlighted the fact that many illnesses are preventable, and that all nurses need to be able to *help people to promote their own health* (DH, 2006a). Nurses can be very influential in promoting 'positive health behaviour' but need to understand about compliance, concordance and adherence, the factors that affect non-adherence and the strategies that enhance adherence. First we will explore the terminology.

There is an ongoing debate regarding the terms used to describe the behaviour of patients following prescribed medication. Many professionals use the terms inter-changeably, but there are key differences.

Compliance to a treatment derives from Latin, meaning 'to complete an action or fulfil a promise'. This could apply to the behaviour desired of the patient. However, to some the word carries a negative connotation implying that patients are passive recipients of treatment, submissive to the power of the professional and conforming to the treatment. Non-compliance is linked to blaming the patient for not following the advice and instructions of the professional.

Concordance to treatment was proposed as an alternative term, suggesting equality and negotiation in the treatment process between the professional and the patient. Using this term can also lead to problems, as some patients do not want or are unwilling to make decisions about their treatment. A further difficulty in using this term is that it is based on the relationship between the professional and the patient and does not necessarily reflect the patient's medicine-taking behaviour. The patient and the professional may have a very positive relationship but external influences such as opinions and information provided by family, friends, media and other patients may impact on their medicine-taking behaviour. Patients may be unwilling to discuss others' attitudes to their medication.

Adherence is defined by NCCSDO (2005) as: *The extent to which the patient's behaviour matches the agreed recommendations from the prescriber.* This term does carry the connotation of 'sticking' but does not confer a derogatory tone, so 'adherence' will be used within this chapter to discuss a patient's ability to follow a medicine regime in terms of taking the correct dose at the right frequency for the correct duration.

Non-adherence

There are numerous reasons why patients do not follow the prescribed treatment. Non-adherence is an important issue in patient care because the health of a patient who does not take the prescribed medication may not improve; continued symptoms may result in a lower quality of life and possible readmission to hospital, which can be a waste of resources. Non-adherence can be intentional – where the patient decides not to follow the prescribed treatment – or unintentional – usually based on inadequate knowledge, instruction or understanding. The nurse needs to be aware of these problems and attempt to help solve them.

Factors influencing non-adherence

Knowledge

The link between patient knowledge and adherence to a prescribed medicine regime is complex. Many patients claim to need more information about their medication but the association of such knowledge with adherence is not clear: many patients may know how and when to take their medication but are not clear about the expected benefit of taking a particular drug, especially when they are taking more than one medicine for a complex illness. This is not to say that providing information to patients about their medication is unimportant or insignificant; what is important is how the information is given and when.

The information provided needs to be technically accurate and should include an explanation of:

- the medicine;
- the dosage;
- the route, with any limiting instructions such as: avoid alcohol, take with food, take after food, avoid operating machinery and driving;
- the purpose of the medicine;
- the duration of the medicine;
- side effects;
- storage requirements.

Poor communication

We have already recognised earlier in this chapter that communication can be a barrier to effective partnership working, and it can also affect the building of a therapeutic relationship with patients. There is a wealth of information available for nurses on communication skills. Communication is a core skill for nurses as included in the *Essence of care* benchmarks (DH, 2003b).

Nurses can express themselves both verbally and non-verbally and need to be confident in the use of both methods so that information can be effectively conveyed to patients regarding their medications. Communication about medication will be highly individualised and adapted to the specific needs of the patient. You need to plan your interaction with the patient and be able to convey the detailed information listed above. You need to ensure that the patient receives consistent advice. Patients with complex illness may encounter a number of health professionals and attend a number of clinics; if information is not consistent between professionals, this will only serve to confuse them. They will wonder who is providing the correct information and possibly decide that if professionals cannot agree, it cannot matter.

The information you provide needs to be succinct because if you give too much information, it will not be retained or recalled with accuracy. You need to be able to use open questions rather than closed questions to elicit the most information from the patient. Patients who are given the opportunity to ask questions appear to be more adherent with their prescribed medicines than those not provided with the opportunity to ask. In line with the RCGP (2009) guidance you need to consider the way the information is best relayed to the particular patient. You can consider using pictures and diagrams to aid your explanations, and if a foreign language poses a potential barrier, then organising an interpreter and providing written information in an alternative language would be to your advantage. You also need to consider any disability that may impact on the effectiveness of your interaction and make adjustments to compensate for this.

Complexity of treatment

With advancing technology and progress in research many patients now receive complex treatment packages. It would appear possible that the more complex the treatment, the greater the potential for non-adherence. Evidence reported by Claxton et al. (2001) suggests that non-adherence increases the more frequently a medicine is required to be taken – for example, a medicine taken three times a day as compared to once or twice a day. Nurses need to be aware of the preparations available for certain drugs, as selecting a longer-acting agent that requires fewer doses may help with adherence.

Prolonged treatment

When patients have prolonged treatment regimes, such as are required for treating epilepsy, diabetes mellitus and asthma, other factors also feature and can affect adherence. For instance, an authoritarian style of interaction can negatively influence adherence. You need to adopt a non-judgemental and non-confrontational approach to medicine taking, especially if you are going to be seeing a patient regularly over many years.

Cost of medication

The expense of prescriptions may stop patients from taking up a prescription or paying for a repeat prescription. In 2010 the cost of a prescription is £7.20 in England. Prescriptions are free from charge in Wales and Northern Ireland and will become free in Scotland in 2011.

Although the cost may be prohibitive, it is usually influenced by other contributing factors such as the severity of the symptoms and illness as perceived by the patient. You may need to tell patients in England that certain medicines are free of charge, such as contraceptives and medicines used in the treatment of tuberculosis (TB) and sexually transmitted diseases. There is also no charge for medicines during pregnancy or for a patient who has been pregnant within the last 12 months, for patients in receipt of certain state benefits including jobseeker's allowance, income support or for patients who are over 60 years of age, although this latter exemption may change with an increase in the retirement age.

Patients with specific diseases can qualify for a medical exemption certificate so they do not have to pay for their medicines. These include illnesses such as cancer, diabetes and epilepsy. You can tell patients who do not qualify for free prescriptions that it may be more cost-effective to buy a Prescription Prepayment Certificate. The price in 2010 is £104 for 12 months or £28.25 for three months.

Inconvenient medicine schedule

We have seen that the number of doses a patient needs to take will affect adherence, so you can help the patient to devise a personal routine on how to incorporate the medicines into their existing daily routine. Of particular importance can be finding a way to help patients to remember to take medications while at work or to work out when to take drugs that can have a fairly rapid response, such as diuretics.

Adolescents and adherence

A number of investigators have found that adolescents experience non-adherence, particularly when they have long-term conditions such as epilepsy, asthma and diabetes mellitus. This can be influenced by normal psychological development: most adolescents strive for independence and a young adult with a long-term illness will dislike both the illness and their dependency on treatment. You can help by being a good listener, giving frank and full information, and by being non-judgemental.

Culture

There is an association between certain cultures and adherence. Asian cultures can be sceptical of modern medicines, preferring more traditional treatments (Horne et al., 2004), and first-generation Caribbean patients have been found to distrust anti-hypertensive agents (to reduce blood pressure), preferring to take medicines only when they feel they need them (Connell et al., 2005). The precise influence of culture on non-adherence is difficult to determine; language is an important factor in adhering to prescribed medication, and this may be the inhibitory factor rather than an individual's cultural background.

Side effects

Nurses have a role to play in monitoring for both the effectiveness of the medicine you have given and the potential side effects.

Many professionals can be confused in relation to the ethics and practicalities of discussing side effects with a patient.

Questions arise such as:

- Should we discuss all of the side effects listed for a particular medicine when some of the reports demonstrate that certain side effects are very rare?
- Does discussing the potential side effects of a medicine have a negative effect on patient adherence as the discussion has perturbed them?

In answer to these questions it is suggested that the most common side effects are discussed, because patients are more likely to stop taking medicines if they are not told of the potential side effects. The most common side effect will be the first one listed on the manufacturer's guidance leaflet. Of particular concern is the situation where a patient is taking multiple medicines, because they may attribute a side effect to the wrong medicine and stop taking the most important medicine, which may not be the one causing that specific side effect.

It is therefore important to educate patients in what to do in the event of experiencing side effects. Some side effects will resolve over time, so the medicine can be continued; other medicines will need to be stopped. So the advice patients should be given is that if side effects occur, they should seek guidance from those who are suitably qualified to make this judgement and provide advice.

Strategies to enhance adherence

Before you venture to address an issue of adherence with a patient you should be assured of the suitability of the medicine prescribed. If a patient is taking an inappropriate medicine, then it will be wasteful in both time and resources because the medicine will have no effect on the underlying illness or symptoms and could lead to unwanted side effects.

You need to ensure that you have accurate knowledge about the benefits of taking the prescribed medicine as well as details on the route of administration, the dose and the frequency the medicine should be taken so that you can convey this information to the patient. Many patients can and do take their medicines appropriately in the hospital setting, but non-adherence can arise following discharge home. They may have unclear instructions as to how long the medicine should be continued, and fail to collect a repeat prescription when necessary. Such information can be written down for the patient on discharge, informing them of how many days of medication are provided by the pharmacy department, and when they will need to organise a repeat prescription if required. Many GP surgeries require a period of notice before collection of a repeat prescription so it may help the patient if you can help them to work out which day the repeat prescription would need to be arranged.

Some patients do not take their medicine correctly as they cannot read the labels on the bottles or cannot open the packaging or the container the medicine is supplied in. You need to assess the manual dexterity of the patient as many have disorders, such as a stroke or arthritis, that reduce manual dexterity and may result in them having difficulty opening certain types of packaging or containers.

You also need to have a working knowledge of the devices available to make the access to medication easier, such as multi-compartment tablet dispensers.

Since 2005 it has been a statutory requirement for the name of a medicine and the strength to be displayed in Braille on the medicine box. Using Braille does not usually apply to injections, but Braille does have to be included on insulin and kidney dialysis fluids as a number of patients receiving these treatments have a visual impairment. This is beneficial to the patient who can read Braille, but may not be the solution for other visually impaired patients. Those who develop visual impairment as a consequence of advancing age may not read Braille, which is a skill mostly acquired by those individuals who have been blind from birth.

Because of the complex names some medicines are attributed, patients often have difficulty in remembering the name and dose of a medicine, and this can result in non-adherence. Confusion and impaired memory can be a feature of a number of illnesses including dementia, HIV infection, liver disease and renal disease. Because brand names are more familiar to some patients, they remember the brand name rather than the generic name. Some patients distinguish medicines by the colour of the medicine and the number they are required to take. This method of recognition has its limitations: you need to warn the patient that the same medicine from different manufacturers can have a different brand name and can come in different strengths.

Scenario

Your patient requires 100mg of her medicine and is usually supplied with 100mg tablets, so she has become accustomed to taking only one tablet. When she is away on a visit, another pharmacist dispenses 50mg tablets and your patient is therefore at risk of being under-dosed. Because you know the medicine comes in different strengths, you have avoided this problem by explaining clearly that this is the case, and that two 50mg tablets add up to the 100mg dose.

Simplicity and importance seem to be the main influences to aid memory, so being able to convey information about medicines in an understandable and memorable fashion is a core skill for nurses as well as being able to stress the significant information to be retained.

We have already mentioned holistic care of our patients in the context of meeting all the patient's needs, whether they be physical, psychological, emotional or spiritual, but the principles of holistic care in relation to medicines requires thought from you as the student nurse in relation to health promotion and lifestyle advice. Some individuals have religious or cultural beliefs that do not promote adherence to the pharmaceutical treatment regimes that are prescribed, and you may wish to pursue other avenues of treatment by using different therapies.

In Chapter 2 we discussed a patient's capacity to consent and the fact that as long as they are aware of the risks and benefits of non-compliance to medication, then their wishes should be respected. As nursing advocates for our patients, our decisions for the care we deliver are based on the patient's best interests; however, this may not necessarily match up with what the patient wants, and we have to respect this.

The story does not end there, however. Our senses are our best tools in nursing: we observe and we assess our patients, and if our patient does not want to receive pain relief, we consider alternatives, starting with the simplest strategies such as helping our patients re-position themselves, providing supporting pillows or other aids. With children a lot of distraction techniques are used, and we could learn from this in adult nursing by improving the environments for our patients; a well-placed picture on the wall or a discussion about the photographs surrounding the patient do not take great resources to achieve but may have a beneficial impact on the patient.

Complementary and alternative therapies

Some patients may enquire about **complementary and alternative therapies**, requiring advice and guidance. In Chapter 4 we discussed the Department of Health document *Extending professional and occupational regulation* (DH, 2009), which identified the recommendation from the Health Professions Council that healthcare groups including traditional Chinese medicine practitioners and herbal medicine practitioners should be statutorily regulated. This move is in the interest of public safety, which should alert us to the fact that alternative and complementary therapies require knowledgeable and competent practitioners to deliver them. In the same way, we are accountable for our practice and the advice we give. Merely experiencing a therapy for yourself or having a family member who approved of the therapy they received is not a basis for knowledge. Successful training must be undertaken by a registrant who wishes to practise these therapies, and in doing so or advising a patient of such therapies the registrant must consider the appropriateness of the therapy in relation to the patient's condition and any treatments they may be receiving. It is also wise to know where the boundaries of vicarious liability are with complementary and alternative therapies to ensure that you as the registrant are not exposed to litigation.

Good record keeping is essential to inform all other healthcare professionals of the therapies that are co-existing with the medical treatments, as the care of the patient may need changing to accommodate the different therapies.

C H A P T E R S U M M A R Y

Inter-professional working is at times complex, with no simple or quick-fit solutions to ensure its success. All team members have a role to play – both individually and as part of the team. There may be barriers that prevent the progression of inter-professional working, for example ineffective communication and a constant use of jargon, but there are also strategies to overcome some of those barriers that need not be complicated but nevertheless require effort. It is important to remember that when we strip away the professional and patient label, underneath we have a person. Every person has feelings and anxieties but needs to be listened to and treated with respect, and that should be central to what we do.

It was the intention of this chapter to highlight the importance of patient centrality within inter-professional working and of positioning the patient's needs above all others. Building a therapeutic relationship is crucial but requires certain key elements, and although communication and inter-personal skills feature highly, so do empathy and genuineness. Nursing is truly an art that requires a medley of skills, none of which should be practised without a rationale or without thought. Consider always how you would feel if you were the patient, or if you had no nursing background: what information would you want and what education would you require? All patients are individuals and should be treated as such. Medicines administration is also an individual aspect of care, which requires the nurse to think about individual needs, whether it be information about medicines and their side effects, help with adherence, or advice surrounding alternative and complementary therapies. As advocates we ensure our patients receive the optimum care and that they remain safe while in our care and when they are at home, which includes ensuring they take their medicines on time and safely. It is important to remember that all health professionals and non-professionals have an important part to play in helping the patient achieve this.

Activities: brief outline answers

Activity 6.1: Team working (page 134)

What actions do you take? You do not administer the 'flush' but excuse yourself from Mrs Wood – explaining you will be back shortly – and follow Dr Williams so that you can explain your actions.

What rationale do you have to support the decisions you have made? You tell Dr Williams that you are unable to 'flush the cannula' because this means you are administering medicines intravenously, which you have not been educated to do. You refer to Standard 20, which states: *Wherever possible two registrants should check medication to be administered intravenously, one of whom should also be the registrant who then administers the IV medication.*

You also identify that even if you had the skill to administer the 'flush', you did not see what was in the syringe as Dr Williams prepared it himself. Standard 14 clearly states: *Registrants must not prepare substances for injection in advance of their immediate use or to administer medication drawn into a syringe or container by another practitioner when not in their presence.*

If Dr Williams cannot administer the 'flush' himself, he should delegate the job to a registrant (qualified nurse) who is suitably skilled.

What could the consequences of your actions be? Standard 18 states: *Students must never administer/supply medicinal products without direct supervision.* It is not enough merely to acknowledge your limitations: you must ensure that the cannula is flushed by an appropriate registrant to ensure the cannula remains patent so that Mrs Wood's treatment can continue safely without discomfort.

Knowledge review

Now that you have completed this chapter, how would you rate your knowledge of the following topics?

	Good	Adequate	Poor
1. The barriers to working inter-professionally and the strategies that can overcome those barriers			
2. The factors that can enhance adherence			
3. The factors that influence non-adherence			
4. The roles and responsibilities of some healthcare workers involved in medicines management			
5. The communication and interpersonal skills to optimise patient medicine taking			

Where you're not confident in your knowledge of a topic, what will you do next?

Further reading

Clothier Report (1994) *Independent inquiry relating to deaths and injuries on the children's ward at Grantham and Kesteven General Hospital.* London: HMSO.

Laming Report (2003) *The Victoria Climbié inquiry:* London: HMSO.

Smith Report (2005) *The Shipman Inquiry:* London: HMSO.

All three reports highlight the importance of team working and communication between services including the health service.

Useful websites

www.dh.gov.uk The website of the Department of Health, which provides information on supplementary prescribing at: **www.dh.gov.uk/prod_consum_dh/groups/dh_digitalassets/@dh/@en/documents/digitalasset/dh_4068431.pdf** (accessed 29 March 2010).

www.parkinsons.org.uk The website of Parkinson's UK, which has information on the 'Get it on time' campaign for people with Parkinson's disease at **www.parkinsons.org.uk/about_us/policy_and_campaigns-1/campaigns/get_it_on_time_campaign/campaign_background.aspx** (accessed 28 March 2010).

www.rpsgb.org.uk The website of the Royal Pharmaceutical Society of Great Britain. The *Code of Ethics for Pharmacists and Pharmacy Technicians* is available at **www.rpsgb.org.uk/pdfs/coeppt.pdf** (accessed 30 March 2010).

Chapter 7

Evidence-based practice

Sarah Ratcliffe and Melanie Stephens

Chapter aims

After reading this chapter, you will be able to:

- understand the importance of evidence-based practice in medicines management;
- understand the evidence behind medicine discovery, development, therapeutic index and evaluation;
- search for up-to-date evidence in order to manage medicines safely in a variety of situations;
- read and evaluate evidence in order to manage medicines safely.

Introduction

Between 2006 and 2009 there were 21,383 patient safety incidents related to delay in administering medicines, 68 resulting in severe harm and 27 in death. One of those deaths was a patient who was admitted with:

> [an] infected ulcer and cellulitis. At 15.00hrs the doctor treating the patient instructed the nurse to give intravenous antibiotics immediately. The doctor returned at 16.30hrs. Observations had not been done and antibiotics not given. Patient was drowsy. Nurse in charge said she was too busy to listen. Staff nurse took manual blood pressure: 70/40, patient tachycardic. Patient had to go to Intensive Care Unit, where she died from severe sepsis.
>
> (NPSA, 2010)

Medicine doses are omitted or delayed in hospital for a variety of reasons. Yet nurses and other healthcare professionals failed on this occasion to realise that these reasons are safety issues and contravene best practice (National Reporting and Learning Service, NPSA, 2009b).

Activity 7.1   *Decision-making*

Imagine you are on the ward where this death occurred. What reasons might the nurse have given to support her decision for not giving the medication? Would any of these reasons you noted be supported in a court of law or at a Nursing and Midwifery Council hearing? What decision should this nurse have taken and why?

An outline answer is given at the end of the chapter.

Decision making in medicines administration and management requires nurses to use their clinical judgement. These judgements are based on many sources of evidence and require personal understanding of the necessary knowledge, skills and attitudes to ensure safe practice.

Evidence in relation to medicines management can include the more obvious sources of information such as the *British National Formulary*, the *Children's British National Formulary*, local policy and guidelines. However, it is imperative that nurses also use less obvious sources such as legislation, NMC guidance, **peer reviewed** articles and expert opinion. Central to all these valuable sources of evidence are the patient and their experience, which, when evaluated collectively, enhance both knowledge and under-standing of medicines management.

What is evidence-based practice?

Since the introduction of the Modernisation Agenda (DH, 1997), practice within the National Health Service has been subject to quality standards and control. A method of ensuring excellence in service delivery is the utilisation of best available evidence. Historically, practice was based on rituals and opinion (Walsh and Ford, 1989), but to ensure that services were driven by continuous quality improvement, the Labour government stated that healthcare in the twenty-first century would be effective in relation to cost, time and resources and that a more robust system of evaluation was needed based on a clear rationale and on evidence. This would affect all aspects of care, including medicines management.

According to Sackett et al. (1996, pp71–2) evidence-based practice (EBP) is *the conscientious, explicit and judicious use of current best evidence in making decisions about the care of individual patients, and involves integrating individual clinical expertise with the best available clinical evidence from research findings.*

For example, in medicines management patients with long-term non-specific back pain were historically advised to rest and take regular analgesia and only if necessary were they referred for physiotherapy. However, on the basis of new evidence, the National Collaborating Centre for Primary Care (2009) proposes the use of a holistic assessment and diagnostic framework. The management of this group of patients currently encompasses many treatment strategies, including structured exercise programmes, self-referral pathways, psychological care and both traditional and complementary forms of pain relief. Rather than reaching for the bottle of painkillers, patients are encouraged to become active recipients of care and experts in the management of their condition (DH, 2001).

Guidelines, policy and legislation require regular **systematic review**; therefore, evidence gathering is a cyclical process and requires consideration of new and current evidence in light of new technologies, practices and patient feedback. A typical view of the process of evidence-based practice is seen in Figure 7.1.

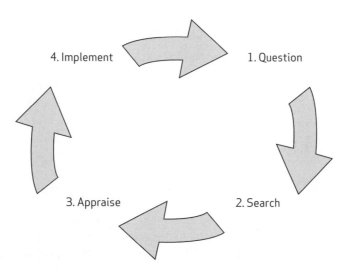

Figure 7.1: Evidence-based practice cycle

Evidence-based practice in relation to medicines management

In order to understand evidence-based practice in medicines management we need first to be sure what we mean by medicines management. The Audit Commission (2001, p5) defines medicines management as *the entire way that medicines are selected, procured, delivered, prescribed, administered and reviewed to optimise the contribution that medicines make to producing desired outcomes of patient care.* The definition from Sackett et al. (1996) above is also helpful. (**Procurement** is defined in the Glossary.)

So evidence-based practice in relation to medicines management can best be defined as the use of current best evidence from a wide range of sources, which involves **critical appraisal**, professional judgement and patient preference (see Figure 7.2).

Evidence-based practice can have an impact on medicines management at every stage of the process, from when the medicine or regime is chosen, purchased and prescribed, to when it is administered and later evaluated. This is the process that you as a nurse must follow when practising evidence-based medicines management:

- identify a problem and turn it into a question;
- carry out a systematic search of the evidence;
- appraise the evidence against a critical appraisal framework.

You should then be able to apply the evidence in keeping with patient preference and evaluate from both a professional and a patient perspective.

For example, in wound care and medicines management, larvae therapy is considered as a cost-effective way to debride sloughy, purulent, infected acute and chronic wounds (Steenvoorde et al., 2007). In order to introduce maggot therapy as a wound-care management option for patients, nurses have to consider the evidence prior to any clinical decisions being made.

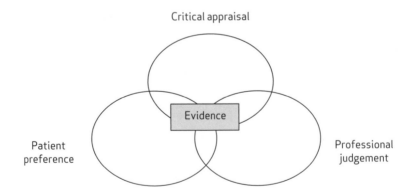

Figure 7.2: The way evidence is framed in practice

Activity 7.2	Decision-making

Imagine you are in a community leg ulcer clinic and treating a patient who has a purulent, infected wound caused by a pre-tibial laceration. What are the issues you need to deal with? How do you apply the procedure described above at each stage of medicines management?

Here are the questions you might ask at each stage:

- *Selection* Why choose maggots? What evidence is there on their use, and how recent, valid and reliable is this evidence?
- **Procurement** How much do the maggots cost in comparison to other wound-care products? How do they compare in effectiveness of removing slough and infection? How quickly do they work?
- *Delivery* How and where will they be delivered? How will they be stored? How much does this cost?
- *Prescription* Are they available on prescription? Who can prescribe them? Are they a medicine or medical device?
- *Administration* What knowledge and skills are required for the safe administration of maggots? Are there any contraindications in the use of larvae therapy?
- *Review* How will the maggot therapy be assessed for its clinical effectiveness (cost, time and audit)?

By generating and answering these questions individual nurses are contributing to the maintenance of clinical effectiveness. Clinical effectiveness is an important aspect of evidence-based practice as nurses have a responsibility to avoid wasting time, effort, money and resources on treatments that have no therapeutic benefit (Alderson and Groves, 2004).

The process from selection to review can also be influenced by factors other than evidence-based guidelines. For example, although evidence suggests that maggot therapy is a worthwhile intervention in wound-care management, best practice may still be hindered for the following reasons.

- Maggot therapy is less likely to be prescribed and used by those who have little knowledge, confidence and experience of wound care and the use of maggots in this field of practice.
- The patient may be put off by the 'yuk' factor (Parnés and Lagan, 2007) of larvae and decline their use.
- The local Trust may not have maggots as part of their wound-care formulary, and maggots may be considered too costly in relation to other dressing products available. The larvae may not be available when the practitioner requires them.

The current body of evidence (National Prescribing Centre, 2009b) suggests that medicines management needs to be continually developed. This can be considered from varying perspectives, for example patient safety, service efficiency and cost.

Evidence-based medicines management: patient safety

Patient safety within medicines management is vital. Safe medicines management can help reduce the likelihood of medication errors and hence patient harm. To ensure the safer administration of medicines, general recommendations have been provided from both the NMC (2007) and DH (2004), and these embrace what can be called 'the five Rs': right patient, right drug, right dose, right route, right time.

For example, when you are working on the ward and carrying out medicines administration it is your responsibility to make the following checks.

1. The name band of the patient corresponds correctly with the drug prescription chart.

2. The correct drug is given to the patient. Check that the drug is correctly prescribed and signed by the initial prescriber on the prescription chart, and has been dispensed in the correct container, for example bottle, box or vial.
3. Prior to administering the medication, it is imperative you check the dose is correct and will be of therapeutic value. This often means you have to check the weight of the patient (clearly labelled on the prescription chart) against the dose. Always refer to the BNF or Children's BNF if you are unsure of the drug or dosage.
4. Check that the correct route has been clearly documented on the prescription chart by the initial prescriber, for example oral, rectal, intramuscular. Then check that the patient can actually receive the drug via the route prescribed.
5. It is then important to check the time that the drug should be given on the prescription chart and how often it should be given in a 24-hour period. This will also include if it should be given at the same time each day or as a 'one-off' dose of medication.

These are the basic checks you must do in every case. However, there are a further three 'rights' that you need to think about.

- *Right assessment* Take into consideration the age of the patient, any allergies, blood or microbiology test results, any underlying medical condition(s) and contraindications of other medication. You may need to make any essential clinical observations before administration of the medication, for example it may be necessary to take the patient's pulse prior to administering digoxin. Informed consent to administer the medication is then gained.
- *Right response* Monitor the effectiveness of the medication administered and observe for the effect and any side effects. For example, has the patient's pain been relieved and their pain score reduced and documented accordingly? During this time, support the patient to concord with the medication regime.
- *Right documentation*   You must correctly mark on the Patient Medicines Administration Chart whether the patient has taken or been given the medication. If you note any adverse effects, these are documented not only in the nursing notes but also in the medical notes, and you must complete an adverse drug reaction form (yellow card, BNF or CBNF). If there is any adverse drug reaction you must communicate with the relevant members of the multidisciplinary team, in a timely and appropriate manner.

By maintaining and following this process in the administration of medicines you are providing quality care and placing best evidence in context with the needs of the patient and the organisation in which you are employed.

Evidence-based medicines management: service efficiency

Within evidence-based medicines management nurses are encouraged to develop innovative and efficient ways of delivering and managing care. Service efficiency is therefore about establishing the least costly solution to address a particular problem or use current resources in the most beneficial way. A recent example from nursing practice and the administration of medicines is the red tabard system proposed within the Productive Ward document (NHSIII, 2008). This involves the nurse wearing a red tabard when undertaking the medicines administration round. The tabard clearly identifies the nurse's role and responsibility on the shift and prevents unnecessary interruptions from other members of staff and patients. The implementation of this change in service promotes efficiency in reducing the number of potential drug errors and has an impact on reducing the length of time a medication round may take.

Evidence-based medicines management: cost

Within the NHS financial pressures are progressively more central to the decisions made by all healthcare staff. In relation to medicines management providers of care need not only to explore what is best for the patient and the organisation, based on the best available evidence, their expertise and patient preference, but also the cost of the medicine or treatment.

Within Nottingham City Hospital the introduction of the Patient's Medicine Bag has led to the reduction in:

- number of faxes to pharmacy about patient medication requirements;
- nursing and other support time spent on searching for information about a patient's medication;
- the number of medications being missed during administration;
- medicines clinical incidents;
- calling others to help with bringing patients' medication in from home;
- expenditure, as £7,389 was saved in the reduction in the use of pharmacy paper bags.

The bag was designed specifically for patients to keep their medications in while in hospital. They are initially given out by paramedics picking up patients from home and are carried with the patient through their stay in hospital and at discharge. According to the trust, *having the medication all in one place allows an increase in the number of medications coming in with the patients and ensures that the patients were presenting with a full medication history* (NHSIII, 2005).

Activity 7.3	Reflection

Understanding terminology used in evidence-based practice

Before reading on, write down what each of the following terms mean:

- **qualitative research**;
- **quantitative research**;
- clinical trial;
- **reliability**;
- **validity**;
- **statistical significance**;
- data;
- recruits;
- **applicability**;
- **control group**;
- **variable**;
- **hypothesis**;
- **generalisability**.

All these terms are given in the glossary so there is no outline answer at the end of the chapter.

The evidence behind medicine discovery, development, evaluation and regulatory approval

Brief history of medicines discovery

Healthcare professions are always looking for new medicines to treat the many illnesses and diseases that affect the general population in which they treat. However, the discovery of medicines is a lengthy process and is influenced by many factors, including those highlighted by the MHRA (2009, pp1–20):

- *advances in the understanding of human biology and healthcare, such as stem cell research and gene therapy, which help scientists piece together how a disease is caused and what processes in the body are involved;*
- *government treatment priorities – diabetes and heart disease, for example;*
- *an ageing population, among whom diseases, such as Alzheimer's disease and cancer, are more common;*
- *global initiatives, such as those to halt new cases of malaria and HIV infection;*
- *the availability of research funding and sponsorship;*
- *the costs and effectiveness of existing medicines;*
- *chance findings, which shift the focus of research – for example, Viagra was originally developed to relieve the chest pain of heart disease, but during tests, men said it helped them with erectile problems, and it was sub-sequently developed for this purpose instead.*

When exploring the possibility of a new medicine, the initial step of the process is exploring how a disease, illness or infection is caused, followed by the stage of developing medicines that either modify or stop a stage of disease or infection progression. The medicine is then advanced either from a current **compound** or from changes made to the make-up of a medicine already available, or by combining new compounds of medicines. This process is known as targeting in the drug industry. The 'target' is the biological cell, or cellular or molecular structure that the developing medicine is meant to affect.

Once a new medicine has been targeted it is screened and then designed. Screening is the process in which new drugs are tested to assess the ability to modify or interrupt the disease or infection. They are also tested to assess the effect on other stages of disease and infection progression, as this may lead to toxicity and damage to other cellular and molecular structures.

Testing is through varying the strength of the medicines, to see how it reacts with different cells and in different conditions. Compounds that have an effect in these varying situations are called lead compounds.

Once screened, the drug is then studied in relation to its physical and biological properties. This allows the pharmacologists to make predictions of the sorts of chemicals that might fit, and new drugs can develop from these tests.

Medicine: the development cycle

A medicine begins its existence as a chemical matter or composite. Many of these compounds may initially show potential but even after years of development may turn out to be of no therapeutic value. This can be for many reasons, for example, they do not work well or they have too many undesirable side effects.

There are six stages to the development cycle of a medicine.

1. *Discovery*   This is when a medical compound is assessed for the possibility of further development and its chemical structure is detailed. Many drugs arise from plant research and observing medicinal plant use in non-Western cultures. This is known as ethnobotany, which is the study of how people of a particular culture and region make use of indigenous plants. For example, **ethnobotanists** studied plants used by four indigenous groups of native Mexicans. Following laboratory studies some of the chemical structures within the plants were found to have anti-inflammatory properties (Heinrich, 2000), particularly effective in treating gastrointestinal, respiratory and dermatological conditions. Similarly, Sharma and Singh (2002) studied herbal remedies commonly used with indigenous groups in Africa and Asia to treat conjunctivitis.
2. *Pre-clinical research*   Tests are then carried out in the laboratory (*in vitro*) and in living tissue (*in vivo*). Although it may seem that there are a multitude of medicines available, thousands of them never get past this stage.
3. *Clinical trials*   Successful compounds from preclinical research are then used in clinical trials. This means that the chemical matter produced is then tested on people. The number of people increases over a phased and lengthy approach, which can often last for six years.
4. *Marketing authorisation*   The manufacturer applies for a licence from the regulator so that the product can be put on the market to sell.
5. *Monitoring*   Even when a medicine has been licensed, both research and monitoring surrounding the use of the drug continues. This includes issues such as the effectiveness and general safety of the medicine.
6. *Changes in the use of a medicine*   Medicines are sometimes used for different reasons than the original indication, and changes in the use of the medicine can be made. Common medicines whose use has changed include amitriptyline (antidepressant and phantom limb pain), haloperidol (acute psychosis and nausea/emesis) and beta-blockers (hypertension and anxiety disorders).

Medicines and evidence-based practice

Medicines are developed using a quantitative approach to evidence-based practice, and testing is through the process of a phased clinical trial. Within medicines management this usually has four phases, each phase being classed as a separate trial (Pocock, 2004). The process of a clinical trial includes these four phases.

1. The principal investigator first ascertains the medication to be tested. Pilot experiments are performed to develop knowledge of how the clinical trial might proceed. The effectiveness of the medicine will be tested in a clinical trial. Groups often excluded from clinical trials are the elderly, women and children even though they are groups of people who will go on to regularly use the medication in the future.
2. During the clinical trials the medicine is then compared to either an existing treatment or a **placebo** (an inert substance), and the type of patients that might benefit from the medication are identified and then recruited. This is usually with the assistance of consultants who are known for their medical knowledge, research and expertise, and can often be in a variety of sites across the country.
3. In order to recruit patients to a clinical trial the patients must first read and understand the information leaflet and then sign a consent form. Following holistic

assessment, the researchers involved in the trial administer the medicine and then collect data about the patient for a clear and agreed period of time. Data collected can include vital signs, medicine concentration levels in the blood and general improvement in the condition of the patient. For example, in the first ever clinical trial on the effect of vitamin C in the cure for scurvy, James Lind (1747) collected data on the effect of different dietary acidic solutions – vinegar, cider, seawater, two oranges and one lemon in barley water and sulphuric acid – on sailors affected by scurvy. He found those who had the oranges and lemon solution showed dramatic improvements in gum and skin signs and symptoms within about six days.

4. Data collected from a clinical trial is then sent to the principal investigator who will analyse the findings using different statistical tests.

Within medicines management clinical research is usually designed as a randomised, double-blind and placebo-controlled trial. These terms are frequently used in quantitative research and it is important to understand their meaning.

- *Randomised* means that each person who is recruited to the trial is randomly allocated to either the test group or a control group (who do not receive the treatment).
- *Blind* indicates that the recruits do not know if they are taking the trial drug or a placebo.
- **Double-blind** is when the researchers also do not know which treatment is being given to the recruits. This is done to reduce bias or interference with the trial.
- A *double-dummy* design is when all recruits are given both the placebo and the real medication at alternate times during the trial, to reduce bias and the placebo effect.
- *Placebo control* is the use of a dummy pill made of an inert substance, which allows the investigators to separate the effect of the treatment from other factors.

It is important to remember that although these types of trials are seen to be the most reliable and valid in terms of research, they too have their limitations. For example, the number of recruits may be smaller than needed to provide sufficient data for statistical significance, and sponsorship of the research by the drug company can affect publication of results and limit the design of the study in the questions it asks. This kind of research also precludes complementary and alternative therapies, which cannot be 'blinded'.

Once the medicine has been manufactured and licensed, the monitoring of the effect of the drug may also include qualitative data collection that explores the effect of the drug on the well-being of the patient. These types of studies can focus on the person's lived experience of an event, therapy or treatment, which can be explored using a variety of methods such as **focus groups**, storytelling, observations and reflections. An example of such a qualitative study is the research by Bergkvist and Wengstrom (2006) who found that the patient's lived experience of chemotherapy was coping with the intolerable side effect of nausea and vomiting. Although perceived as a common side effect of chemotherapy usually controlled with anti-emetics, Bergkvist and Wengstrom highlight to healthcare practitioners that its management may have an effect on patient's future treatment decisions and their current understanding of their illness. If nausea and vomiting are not successfully dealt with for this group of patients, then issues such as informed decision making could be affected.

Medical devices

Most wound and stoma care products are classified as medical devices and as such have not undergone the rigour of phased clinical trials. They require prescribing under the Medicines Act 1968, but must not be mistaken for medicinal products. Evidence to support the use of these products is derived from case studies, company literature, smal-scale controlled trials and systematic reviews.

Activity 7.4   *Evidence-based practice and research*

An hour after packing a patient's pilonidal sinus with an alginate dressing, on the second occurrence since surgery, you find him slurring his words, pale and sweaty, with a rapid pulse, fast breathing and hypotension. Apart from his sinus, he has no other past medical history. On examination by the medical team and removal of the alginate they diagnose toxic shock syndrome.

What evidence might the medical team have drawn upon to make their diagnosis?

An outline answer is given at the end of the chapter.

Evidence sources for clinical decision making

In order to practise safely within medicines management and the realms of clinical effectiveness it is important that you know about a range of sources of evidence that may help inform your clinical decision making. To help you assess the reliability and validity of these types of evidence you can use a 'hierarchy of evidence' (see Figure 7.3 on page 159) alongside professional judgement and patient preference.

British National Formulary (*and yellow card*)

The *BNF* is published twice a year by the British Medical Association and the Royal Pharmaceutical Society. It is a reference book that contains information and advice on medications that are used within the NHS. It includes information on drug indications, contraindications, doses, side effects and legal classifications. The *BNF* also holds information on the generic names, the proprietary drug names and the prices of the drug. Although the *BNF* makes reference to most drugs used within the NHS it also contains information on medicines that are only available privately. The *BNF* is also available electronically.

Monthly Index of Medical Specialities (*MIMS*)

MIMS was first published in 1957 and continues to be published monthly. It is a pharmaceutical prescribing reference containing information about all drugs in the UK formulary. An electronic version (eMIMS) is also available for use.

National Institute for Health and Clinical Excellence (NICE)

NICE is the independent organisation responsible for providing national guidance on the promotion of good health and the prevention and treatment of ill health. NICE develops and publishes guidance on issues concerning public health, health technologies and clinical practice. NICE guidance is developed using a wide array of evidence, drawing upon the knowledge of experts working within the NHS as well as people from the wider healthcare setting, such as healthcare professionals from many disciplines, patients and carers, industry and experts from the academic world.

National Patient Safety Agency (NPSA)

The NPSA plays an integral part in patient safety and medicines management. Linked to the Department of Health, the NPSA improves patient safety by informing, supporting and influencing organisations and people working within the wider healthcare community. The three main divisions of the NPSA are:

- National Reporting and Learning Service;
- National Clinical Assessment Service;
- National Research Ethics Service.

For example, the NPSA was instrumental in ensuring the safe care and management of enterally fed patients. In addition, it informs healthcare professionals on the risks involved in administering crushed medication via nasogastric and percutaneous feeding tubes. This followed a series of serious events and incidents involving patient deaths.

Non-governmental organisations

NGOs are registered charities and organisations without government participation or representation, but which may receive funding from private pharmaceutical companies. An example is the British Heart Foundation which has Life-Saving Science reports on recent discoveries (BHF, 2009).

Expert patient programmes

There are a range of education programmes that are peer led and develop self-support for patients with long-term conditions, their carers and families. According to the National Primary Care Research and Development Centre, the programmes *develop patients and their significant others' self-belief, knowledge and skills to manage their condition in order to reduce their use of health and social care services* (NPCRDC, 2006). Patients are vital to the gathering of evidence behind medicines management and their stories and voices provide material to help inform and improve practice.

Nursing and Midwifery Council (NMC)

The NMC was established in 2002 after the UKCC and English National Boards were disbanded in 2001. Set up by the UK government, the NMC regulates all nurses and midwives currently working within the UK. Registration to the NMC is mandatory in order to practise as a midwife or nurse. One of the key roles of the NMC is to protect the public. To do this the NMC sets and reviews standards for nursing education, training, conduct and performance. An example of this guidance is the *Standards for medicines management* (NMC, 2007) and the *Guidance on professional conduct for nursing and midwifery students* (NMC, 2009).

Legislation

Medicines manufacture, research and supply are governed by various pieces of legislation, statutory instruments, impact assessments and NHS directives. These include:

- Medicines Act 1968;
- Misuse of Drugs Act 1971;
- Health Act 2006;
- Directions on the Health Service Act 2006;
- impact assessment of new arrangements under Part IX of the Drug Tariff for the provision of stoma, urology and other appliances;
- The Medicines (Pharmacies) (Responsible Pharmacist) Regulations 2008, Statutory Instrument 2008 No. 2789.

The NHS Institute for Innovation and Improvement

This NHS department actively encourages healthcare staff to explore and develop new ways of working, create new technological advances and promote high-quality leadership. Within medicines management new ways of working have been explored and developed; an example from practice is the Clinical Medicine Review Services in Hull PCT, which is a system to help patients with long-term conditions manage their medication (NHSIII, 2009).

The National Prescribing Centre

An NHS-developed organisation, the NPC has a mission to support and advance service delivery and patient care within medicines management. It regularly produces resources and guidance for healthcare professionals.

The Medicines and Healthcare products Regulatory Agency

Another government organisation, the MHRA is accountable for medicines and devices being safe to use. It provides evidence such as safety information, warnings, guidance, consultations and reports.

The Cochrane Collaboration

This organisation appraises and reviews healthcare interventions from randomised controlled trials, known as Cochrane Reviews, that can be found in the Cochrane Library available electronically via the internet. The reviews are produced by volunteers from across the world. Systematic reviews are seen as the gold standard of evidence-based practice.

Pharmaceutical companies

Drug companies often produce or sponsor evidence to support the use of their products in clinical practice. The evidence provided can range from **randomised controlled clinical trials**, controlled clinical trials, cross-over studies, cross-sectional studies, experimental studies, **cohort studies**, case studies and expert opinion.

Care Quality Commission

The CQC was established in 2009, and its role is to regulate and inspect health and social care services in England whether provided by the NHS, voluntary organisations, local authorities or private companies, and including services provided in the patient's own home. Its publications include documents such as corporate publications, surveys, council reports, standards of care reviews and studies.

Department of Health

This division of the UK government has the duty to develop and ensure health and social care policy for England. The Secretary of State for Health is the lead figure head of the department with two Ministers of State and three Parliamentary Under-Secretaries of State. The work of the DH is to develop and establish national standards of practice and guidance that help focus services delivery and management to promote healthier living and care. Documents available from the Department of Health include legislation, white and green papers, statistics, letters, circulars, bulletins, surveys, fact sheets, command papers and annual reports.

Local policy

Within each trust and healthcare organisation there is a set of documents that describe the necessary principles used as a guide for action and a series of actions necessary for the accomplishment of the goal or course of action, commonly known as policies and procedures. In healthcare, policies and procedures are often influenced by governmental regulation.

Journal articles and books

Regularly used to review current practices, journals usually contain primary research describing studies by the original author(s) or reviews that summarise an aspect of service delivery, care or management. Peer reviewed journals contain both primary and secondary sources of evidence and biographies.

Books are considered excellent secondary sources of evidence. They are often peer reviewed and provide good quality information.

Conference papers

Conference papers are presented and discussed at numerous symposiums for researchers, practitioners and academics. These papers provide a significant route for the exchange and discussion of research studies, reviews and evaluations.

Activity 7.5 *Decision-making*

Acute bacterial meningitis requires immediate identification and management as mortality rates are high if it is left untreated. Best practice suggests that appropriate antibiotics should be administered within 30 minutes of presentation, yet research findings show that delays in administration can range from 2 to 4.9 hours (Proulx et al., 2005).

If as a nurse you had to account for such a delay in practice, what evidence could you refer to and of what assistance could it be?

An outline answer is given at the end of the chapter.

Evaluating evidence in order to manage medicines safely

After searching for supportive evidence it is important to be able to effectively appraise the evidence to inform your decision making and also be able to manage medicines safely. The Critical Appraisal Skills Programme (CASP) has developed tools for use by healthcare staff to help with evaluating and reviewing evidence in a systematic way.

As a nurse it is important to be aware of the hierarchies of evidence used to grade research in accordance with the validity of the work (Sackett et al., 1996). Many frameworks centre on clinical effectiveness, and therefore systematic reviews and randomised controlled trials (RCTS) are categorised higher than other pieces of evidence. However, Evans (2002) suggests that even research graded lower than RCTs presents a distinct viewpoint and should be judged on effectiveness, appropriateness and feasibility.

There are many hierarchies of evidence available, but as a nurse you need to find one that you can understand and use to appraise the available information, and that sits comfortably with your research standpoint.

Traditionally in science there have been two types of evidence:

- **primary evidence**: the original studies, based on trials and studies on subjects;
- **secondary evidence**: generally appraisals of published research that extract findings from two or more studies.

These two types of evidence produced by researchers, academics and practitioners are then often ranked in order of robustness. A traditional hierarchy is seen in Figure 7.3.

However, NICE (2006b) suggests that those reviewing evidence for systematic review should move away from the traditional system based upon effectiveness and promote a more rounded approach, questioning cost-effectiveness, new technology development, inappropriate and unacceptable interventions and the feasibility of actually implementing the intervention in clinical practice. This has been taken a step further by GRADE Working Group (Guyatt et al., 2008) who rank evidence by the following criteria.

- *High quality*   Further research is very unlikely to change our confidence in the estimate of effect.
- *Moderate quality*   Further research is likely to have an important impact on our confidence in the estimate of effect and may change the estimate.

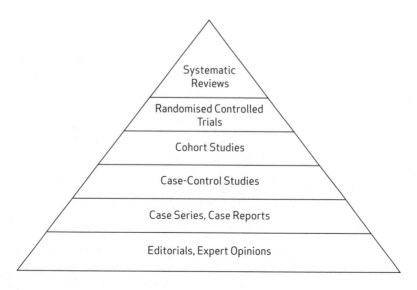

Figure 7.3: A hierarchy of evidence sources

- *Low quality*   Further research is very likely to have an important impact on our confidence in the estimate of effect and is likely to change the estimate.
- *Very low quality*   Any estimate of effect is very uncertain.

Activity 7.6   *Communication*

What is meant by the following types of evidence?

- systematic review;
- randomised controlled trials;
- cohort studies;
- **case control studies**;
- **case series**;
- **case reports**;
- **editorials**;
- expert opinion.

When you are next on a ward round, ask the medical staff why they might choose one type of medicine over another and ask them to provide a rationale for their choice. Then discuss this with the pharmacist. Was there a difference in opinion, and why?

All these terms are given in the Glossary so there is no outline answer at the end of the chapter.

We now look at an example of the way evidence is used in formulating guidelines for best practice.

The advice on crushing tablets

The Nursing and Midwifery Council advises against the crushing of medication for several reasons.

The crushing of medication before administration in most cases renders its use as 'unlicensed'. Consequently, the manufacturers may assume no liability for ensuing harm that may come to the patient or the person administering it. Indeed, the nurse who has administered the crushed medication would be accountable and could be sued for negligence (Griffiths et al., 2003).

Under the Medicines Act 1968, only medical and dental practitioners can authorise the administration of unlicensed medicines to humans. An exception to this is in the case of botulinum toxin. This can be prescribed by supplementary nurse prescribers but only under specific conditions. They can prescribe as part of a clinical management plan that has been agreed in partnership with the independent prescriber (doctor or dentist) and the nurse.

When a medicine is authorised to be administered unlicensed by an independent prescriber, a percentage of liability for any harm that may ensue will still lie with the administering nurse. The balance of this liability would be assessed in a court of law on an individual case basis.

When a medicine is required to be administered via a **PEG tube** (inserted via the subcutaneous tissue of the abdomen into the stomach to provide fluid and nutrition), nurses are advised to discuss the situation with the independent prescriber and the pharmacist. An alternative drug should be used where possible. If there is no option but to crush the medication, then the manufacturer should be contacted to establish whether this is advisable.

Crushing tablets alters the chemical properties of the medication. Schier et al. (2003) report a case in which a crushed, extended-release nifedipine tablet contributed to a patient's death. The patient was administered crushed extended-release nifedipine (a calcium channel blocker) and labetalol (a beta-blocker) via a naso-gastric feeding tube. Both these medications were administered at the same time. The patient developed worsening bradycardia with hypotension and experienced asystolic cardiac arrest. She was resuscitated, but the following morning the same crushed medications were once again administered via the naso-gastric tube. She again developed worsening bradycardia with hypotension and she later died. Although this is a single case study, this evidence does demonstrate that the repeated administration of crushed extended-release nifedipine and labetalol via a naso-gastric feeding tube prevented a compensatory heart rate increase. The release characteristics of controlled-release medications are destroyed when crushed, resulting in the massive bio-availability of the drug amount (see Chapter 4).

Some formulations are enteric coated, which enables them to pass through the upper gastrointestinal tract intact, not releasing the drug until they reach the alkaline environment of the small intestine. Crushing tablets or opening capsules will destroy the protective coat, thus exposing the mucous membranes to potentially irritant active ingredients or resulting in deactivation of acid-sensitive medicines (Kelly et al., 2009).

The issues surrounding the administration of medication via a PEG tube for nurses when it involves the crushing of medication are many and include concerns regarding blockages in the tube. Usually such blockages are caused by previously crushed tablets. One serious potential risk to the patient is that when the nurse tries to remove the blockage by flushing the tube, a bolus of a previously administered medication is inadvertently delivered to the patient.

Authorisation for unlicensed medication administration (crushing of tablets) should always be obtained in writing and not accepted verbally. You must clearly state in the patients' notes the reasons why the medication is being crushed, and communicate the reasons to the patient and the other members of the multidisciplinary team. A care plan should also be implemented to identify this intervention with the reason clearly stated.

Another point for careful consideration is whether the nurse crushing the medication has a sensitivity to the drug concerned. In such cases, even minimal contact with the medication could result in a serious reaction (Kelly et al., 2009).

Complementary and alternative medicines (CAMs)

Over the last 20 years there has been a major increase in interest in **complementary and alternative medicines** (CAMs), from both the general public and health professionals (Mantle and Tiran, 2009). The use of CAMs may result from recommendations by family, friends and the media. Yet there is little research documented in the medical journals reporting their success. This may have led to a lack of information of CAMs within the healthcare professions. Patient choice is central to evidence-based medicines management. As such, the patient should be enabled to utilise CAMs alongside their routine medicine regime if they so wish and if safe to do. However, there is ongoing debate concerning the evidence base that underlies the use of CAMs, and many professionals may be reticent to incorporate CAMs into their practice or to advise patients on their safe use. The healthcare professional has a duty to search for and appraise safe and reliable evidence in order to acquaint the patient with the necessary knowledge to make informed choices about their care. It has been documented that there are often contraindications between CAMs and traditional Western prescribed medicine that the prescriber and drug administrator needs to be aware of. For example, the medicinal herb *Ginkgo biloba* should be avoided in patients that are at risk of bleeding or who are taking anticoagulants (Heyneman, 2003). Ginseng is contraindicated in many psychiatric disorders. Nevertheless, there is an emerging body of evidence reported within the medical journals for other forms of CAMs such as acupuncture for chronic pain relief and St John's Wort for the relief of mild to moderate depression.

Older people and children

Caution is required concerning the medicines management of the more vulnerable patient. Medicines prescribed for children and the older person may not necessarily have been researched on that age group. Reasons for this are many. Because of their vulnerability older people and children are often omitted from clinical drug trials, which often involve complex ethical and policy restraints. In addition, older people tend to have many co-morbidities and poly-pharmacy and may be excluded from clinical trials for these reasons. As a consequence, results from clinical trials are often **extrapolated** to both these groups of patients. Evidence-based practice can therefore be compromised.

Townsley et al. (2005) argue that the lack of older people in the recruitment to clinical trials has revealed a limited knowledge base about the effectiveness of therapies despite the high percentage of prescriptions consumed by older people. Some allude to the divergent characteristics of elderly people in terms of poly-pharmacy and co-morbidities and the potential impact this may have on trial outcomes. Additionally, it is believed that pharmacokinetic and pharmacodynamic changes in the elderly can modify the pharmacologic effect of a drug (Odeh-Ramadam and Remington, 2002). Certainly, it is accepted that the ageing process itself can have a dramatic effect on the rates of drug absorption and bioavailability (Watson, 2000). For example, impaired renal and liver function means that a specific dose of a drug can have a greater effect on an older person's body than on the body of someone younger. (These issues are discussed more fully in Chapter 4.)

Drug calculation formulas

As a nurse it is essential that you are able to competently and correctly work out drug calculations in order to safely administer medicines (NMC, 2007) – see Chapter 1 for a detailed discussion of drugs calculations. Yet literature has highlighted that many nurses and student nurses have a poor standard of skill in this area (Wright, 2006) and that this has led to drug errors and injury to the patient.

The most familiar technique for calculating the prescribed amount of medication is to use the following formula:

$$\frac{\text{What you want}}{\text{What you have}} \times \text{What's it in}$$

Most of the research in this area focuses not on the formula but on the way it is used. When trying to work out the dose needed, the nurse cannot visualise or conceptualise the medication needed and correctly apply the formula to it. Work carried out by Kelly and Colby (2003) found that when student nurses were allowed to work out drug calculations using their own methods of arithmetic and formulas, the calculations were more successful. The main reason for this, according to Wright (2008a), is that the calculation is not meaningful to them and has no direct relevance to the context. It is experienced just as a mathematical equation and not seen as a drug. Add to this confusion a frequent lack of confidence in maths ability, and mistakes can easily occur: the nurse cannot make sense of why each action within the formula is required (Wright,

2007). This may account for the lack of use of the formula in clinical practice as Hoyles et al. (2001) found in their small-scale study of paediatric nurses. Wright (2008b) suggests that the lack of use of the formula in nursing practice is because of the strategy used by the individual nurse to keep the meaning of the numbers current in the equation. Other methods used by nurses include:

- repeat additions and doubling and halving for calculating oral doses;
- compensating, breaking the number down into simple units and building blocks for calculating dosage based on weight;
- 'proportional reasoning' for drugs available by weight and volume; this method looks at the relationship between the drug available as a weight or as a volume, and how much has to be given to make the correct dose.

Activity 7.7   *Evidence-based practice and research*

Access and read the following articles by Wright.

Wright, K (2008a) Drug calculations part 1: a critique of the formula used by nurses. *Nursing Standard*, 22 (36): 40–2.

Wright, K (2008b) Drug calculations part 2: alternative strategies to the formula. *Nursing Standard*, 22 (37): 42–4.

Make notes on the meanings of:

- repeat additions and doubling and halving for calculating oral doses;
- compensating, breaking the number down into simple units and building blocks for calculating dosage based on weight;
- proportional reasoning for drugs available by weight and volume measurements.

Which method makes sense to you?

    Look again at Chapter 1. How does the formula above help with you in developing skill in drugs calculation? If you are still struggling with drug calculations, you must discuss this with your personal tutor and mentors in practice, so appropriate actions and resources can be put in place to help you.

As it is expected that the student will explore which method best suits their own learning style and understanding of drug calculation, there is no outline answer at the end of the chapter.

C H A P T E R   S U M M A R Y

Decision making in medicines administration and management requires nurses to use their clinical judgement. Clinical judgements are based upon critical appraisal, professional judgement and patient preference.

    Evidence-based practice in relation to medicines management is the use of current best evidence from a wide range of sources that involves critical appraisal, professional judgement and patient preference.

    Nurses practising evidence-based medicines management are able to identify a problem and turn it into a question, carry out a systematic search of the evidence, and appraise the evidence against a critical appraisal framework. The nurse should then be able to apply the evidence in keeping with patient preference and evaluate from both a professional and a patient perspective.

Prior to choosing a medicine or wound-care dressing nurses and healthcare practitioners should consider their selection, delivery, prescription, administration and review.

Evidence-based medicines management is based upon three cornerstones of continually developing practice: patient safety, service efficiency and cost.

Patient safety within medicines management is vital, and nurses ought to take into account the 'eight Rs': right patient, right drug, right dose, right route, right time, right assessment, right response and right documentation. Service efficiency is therefore about establishing the least costly solution available to address a particular problem or to use current resources in the most beneficial way.

In relation to medicines management, providers of care need to explore not only what is best for the patient and the organisation, based on the best available evidence, their expertise and patient preference, but also the cost of the medicine or treatment.

There are six stages to the development of a medicine: discovery, pre-clinical research, clinical trials, marketing authorisation, monitoring and changes in the use of a medicine (MHRA, 2009).

Medicines are developed using a quantitative approach to evidence-based practice, and testing is through the process of a phased clinical trial; within medicines management this usually has four phases, each phase being classed as a separate trial.

Once a medicine has been manufactured and licensed, the monitoring of the effect of the drug may also include qualitative data collection that explores the effect of the drug on the well-being of the patient.

Most wound and stoma care products are classified as medical devices and as such have not undergone the rigour of phased clinical trials.

In order to practise safely within medicines management and the realms of clinical effectiveness it is important that an individual nurse has knowledge of the range of sources of evidence that may help inform clinical decision making. These can range from the BNF to legislation, guidelines, policies and journal articles.

There are many hierarchies of evidence available, but nurses need to find one that they can understand and use to appraise the literature.

There will be circumstances when you will find evidence is conflicting; as a practitioner it is imperative to find out your local trust policy guidance, especially in relation to vicarious liability areas, which can include complementary and alternative medicine (CAM), injection technique, older people and children and drug calculation formulas.

Activities: brief outline answers

Activity 7.1: Decision-making (page 146)

Some reasons could be that the ward was too busy or understaffed, that the nurse was waiting for the doctor to prescribe the medicine on the correct drug prescription form, or that the nurse was not aware how unwell the patient was.

These reasons would not be supported in a court of law or at an NMC hearing unless there was adequate evidence to prove that the nurse had followed trust policy and made attempts to improve staffing, or requested the correct prescription of the IV antibiotic. It is the nurse's responsibility to accurately assess the patient's condition and respond appropriately. The nurse should have ensured that the IV antibiotics were administered promptly.

It is important that you refer to the NMC *Standards for medicines management* for a more detailed understanding.

Activity 7.2: Decision-making (page 148)

Issues include patient age and past medical history, patient preference in terms of dressing type or therapy, type of wound, availability of different therapies and wound dressings, local guidelines and policies, and cost. Appraise the quality of the evidence in order to identify the quality and applicability to the patient's condition.

Activity 7.4: Evidence-based practice and research (page 155)

The evidence that the medical team would have drawn upon to make their diagnosis would include: past medical history, investigations, signs and symptoms, previous experience, articles and studies, *BNF*, wound-care company information and pharmacist opinion.

Activity 7.5: Decision-making (page 158)

The four key documents to present in this case would be the nursing notes, Patient Medicines Administration Chart, clinical incident report and off-duty records. The off-duty records would highlight whether the ward was busy and understaffed; it would show the staff–patient ratio and the skill mix on the shift in question. The nursing notes and Patient Medicines Administration Chart have your comments about why you gave the medication late and the reason for the omission. A clinical incident report would be completed as a matter of good practice to highlight that the drug had been given late.

Other documents to include might be any audit of practice within medicines management that had been carried out during the time that the incident occurred, and trust policy documents that would contain specific guidance on the administration of medicines.

Knowledge review

Now that you have completed the chapter, how would you rate your knowledge of the following topics?

	Good	Adequate	Poor
1. The relationship between evidence-based practice and medicines management			
2. The process of selecting a medicine			
3. The development cycle of a medicine			
4. The phases of a clinical trial			
5. The sources of evidence to access in relation to medicines management			
6. The critical appraisal of evidence in medicines management			
7. The conflicting evidence in medicines administration			

Where you're not confident in your knowledge of a topic, what will you do next?

Further reading

British National Formulary (2009) London: BNF.
A biannual publication that includes information on drug indications, contraindications, doses, side effects and legal classifications.

Dougherty, L and Lister, S (2008) *Royal Marsden Hospital manual of clinical nursing procedures*, 7th edition. London: Wiley Blackwell.
A student manual that includes clinical knowledge so that students can be fully informed.

Nursing and Midwifery Council (2008) *Standards for medicines management*. London: NMC.
Sets out guidance for nurses for the safe administration of medicines and medicines management.

Useful websites

www.audit-commission.gov.uk A government organisation that regulates the efficiency of services within the NHS.

www.cochranelibrary.com An organisation that utilises 20,000 experts and academics across the world who review and appraise RCTs; the reviews are then stored on an electronic library.

www.cqc.org.uk An organisation that regulates health and adult social care services in England.

www.dh.gov.uk Website of the Department of Health, whose work is to develop and establish national standards of practice and guidance, which helps focus services delivery and management to promote healthier living and care. Documents available from the DH include papers such as legislation, white and green papers, statistics, letters, circulars, bulletins, surveys, factsheets, command papers and annual reports.

www.institute.nhs.uk A department within the NHS that actively encourages healthcare staff to explore and develop new ways of working, create new technological advances and promote high quality leadership.

www.mhra.gov.uk Provides evidence such as safety information, warnings, guidance, consultations and reports.

www.nice.org.u Develops and publishes guidance on issues concerning public health, health technologies and clinical practice.

www.nmc-uk.org Contains standards for nursing education, training, conduct and performance.

www.npc.co.uk An organisation developed by the NHS whose mission is to support and advance service delivery and patient care within medicines management.

www.npsa.nhs.uk Website of the National Patient Safety Agency, which improves patient safety by informing, supporting and influencing organisations and people working within the wider healthcare community.

Glossary

accountability: giving an account for one's actions and/or omissions.

Act: law made by Parliament also referred to as statute.

actus rea: the physical element of a crime.

advocate: someone who acts on someone else's behalf.

ampoule: a sealed vial which can contain solids or liquids.

antibacterial: medicine used to treat infections caused by bacteria.

anticoagulant: drug that prevents the inappropriate clotting of the blood, used to prevent or reduce clot formation.

applicability: the degree to which research findings are relevant for an area of clinical practice or a phenomenon.

autonomous: with self-determination.

AV: atrioventricular node – part of the conduction system responsible for the beating of the heart. It is composed of specialised nervous tissue situated between the atria and ventricles of the heart.

bioethics: a branch of ethics relating to health technology.

bolus: a single dose of a drug given over a short period of time.

buccal mucosa: the membrane lining the cheeks inside the mouth.

case citation: a way that legal cases are reported.

case control studies: focus on specific populations and events bounded by time.

case law: judge-made law.

case report: a detailed patient report that records symptoms, signs, diagnosis, treatment and follow-up of an individual patient. Case reports may contain a demographic profile of the patient, but usually describe an unusual or novel occurrence.

case series: a method of research that examines medical records to gain an understanding of the relationship between intervention and outcome.

causation: defines the requirement for there to be liability in negligence.

claimant: the person bringing the claim within a civil case.

clinical effectiveness: the method by which optimum benefits of treatments and management are appraised, planned, delivered and reviewed.

clinical trial: a study to test the effectiveness and safety of a drug, technology or procedure.

cohort study: a type of longitudinal study involving a group or groups of people who have the same condition, and observes the effect of an intervention on those who receive it compared to those who do not.

complementary and alternative therapies/complementary and alternative medicine (CAM): alternative approaches to Western biomedicine that often utilise therapies from a cultural or historical basis. Examples include acupuncture, homeopathy, traditional Chinese medicine, herbalism and hypnosis. If used instead of conventional therapies, these treatments are alternative; if used alongside conventional medical treatments, they are complementary.

compliance: derives from Latin, meaning 'to complete an action or fulfil a promise'; applies to the behaviour desired of the patient.

compound: a chemical substance that contains two or more chemical elements.

concordance: an alternative term to compliance, suggesting equality and negotiation in the treatment process between the professional and the patient.

consent: approval or assent.

consequentialism: an approach that considers that the value of an action whether it is right or wrong is based on the consequences of the action.

contraindication: factors that increase the risks involved in using a particular drug.

control group: the group of test subjects left untreated or unexposed to some procedure and then compared with treated subjects in order to validate the results of the test.

criminal actions: or omissions have to be heard in a criminal court; the remedy is prosecution and sanction.

critical appraisal: the process of carefully and systematically examining research to judge its trustworthiness, and its value and relevance in a particular context.

damages: the compensation awarded in civil cases.

data: a record of observations made during the research project, either qualitative or quantitative.

decimal: (decimal fraction) part of a whole number. A decimal point is used to show which place value column each digit needs to appear in. For example, in the number 2.4 there are two whole numbers and 4 tenths of a whole number.

defendant: the person a civil case is brought against.

deontology: an ethical theory where the moral rule has to be followed by all and imposes a duty on us.

dependent prescriber: professionals who are authorised to prescribe certain medicines for patients whose condition has been diagnosed or assessed by an independent prescriber, within an agreed assessment and treatment plan (DH).

digit: an individual numeral. For example, 4 is a digit, as is 5. An example of a 2-digit number would be 23 or 87.

dilemma: where a difficult choice has to be made between competing options.

distribution: the process of how the absorbed drug is circulated around the body, delivering a drug to the site of action.

double-blind: a design in which both the subjects and the researchers are unaware of which drug each group is receiving.

dpm: drops per minute. This relates to the rate of flow for intravenous delivery of medicines.

editorial: an opinion piece written by the senior editorial staff or publisher of a nursing journal.

egoism: an approach whereby individual moral agents do what is in their own self-interest.

enteral route: one using the gastrointestinal tract for the absorption of the drug into the body including oral, sublingual, buccal and rectal routes; the manufacturer will produce drug preparations suitable for using these structures for absorption.

enteric coated: preparations designed to have an acid-resistant covering so they are not dissolved or destroyed by stomach acid; they should not be crushed or chewed when given to the patient.

enzymes: proteins that catalyse specific chemical reactions in the body.

ethical dilemma: a dilemma where you have to make a choice out of two possible solutions, neither of which you feel comfortable with. For example, you are working in intensive care and news comes to you that there has been a major disaster. One victim has multiple injuries and requires intensive care but chances of survival are slim. Another victim has injuries that are serious but not life threatening. You have one bed left. The dilemma is: who should get the bed?

ethics: wherein a community expresses its values.

ethnobotanist: a person who studies the complex relationship between cultures and their use of indigenous plants.

excretion: the process a drug will go through to be eliminated from the body.

expert opinion: thoughts and opinions of a knowledgeable practitioner who is considered a specialist within their field of practice.

extrapolation: using facts and data to draw conclusions about something that is unknown.

fidelity: strict adherence to truth or facts.

fiduciary: entrusting yourself to another.

focus group: a research approach that asks the respondents about their perceptions, opinions, beliefs and attitudes towards a service or treatment. Questions are asked in an interactive group setting where participants are free to talk with other group members.

fraction: a part of a whole number. The bottom number (denominator) shows how many equal parts the whole had been split into, and the top number (numerator) shows how many of those parts we have. For example, 2/5 or two-fifths means that the whole has been split into five equal parts, and we have two of them.

generalisability: the characteristic of research findings that allow them to be applied to other situations or populations.

generic name: the commonly used name of a drug that is not a brand name.

holistic: from the Greek (*holos*) meaning whole, complete or total, it refers in healthcare to treating a patient in mind, body and soul rather than just someone with a physical illness.

hypothesis: a statement that is challenged or verified by observation and investigation.

independent prescriber: *professionals who are responsible for the initial assessment of the patient and for devising the broad treatment plan, with the authority to prescribe the medicines required as part of that plan* (DH).

INR: International Normalised Ratio – a blood test used to monitor patients receiving anticoagulation medicines. This standard international system has been developed as there was a wide variation between different hospitals and different countries in the measurement of the effectiveness of anticoagulant therapies.

intravenous: administered directly into a vein.

involuntary manslaughter: where the defendant did not have the *mens rea* to carry out an act.

judicial precedent: an application to the Supreme Court for a judicial or administrative decision to be reviewed.

legislation: the making or giving of laws by an authority, such as the government Department of Health.

liability: something that someone is responsible for.

lipoatrophy: degeneration of fat tissue in the skin usually as a result of poor sub-cutaneous injection technique.

lipohypertrophy: overgrowth of fat tissue in the skin, usually a reaction in the skin experienced by incorrect injection technique.

meniscus line: the curved shape of fluid within a container. The word meniscus is based on the Greek word for crescent shaped. When measuring medicines, the lower meniscus line must be read at eye level for accuracy.

mens rea: the mental element of a crime.

metabolism: the process by which a drug will be deactivated and prepared for excretion by the kidneys.

moral distress: where the appropriate and ethical action does not take place, for example, where patients are treated aggressively with medication, say for a terminal illness, when it is understood there is no benefit.

moral obligation: an act that is viewed as having value by others; so we may say we have a moral obligation to be honest because society regards it as valuable.

necrosis: cell death. The word is derived from the Greek *nekros* meaning dead body. Cells can die from a number of adverse events such as exposure to toxins, excessive cold or an insufficient blood supply.

nephrotoxic: toxic to the kidney, which is mainly responsible for the removal of drugs from the body.

neurotransmitter: a compound produced and released by activated nerve cells that can cross the distinct physical gap (synapse) in the nerve fibre, gland or muscle, which will respond to the neurotransmitter signal.

nociceptors: sensory nerve fibres for pain perception, located in the skin and organs of the body and detect tissue damage, relaying the signal to the spine and brain.

non-medical prescribing: undertaken by professionals who are not medically trained but who have undertaken a recognised programme of education to be registered to prescribe medicines from a formulary.

normative ethics: a means of comparing values of right and wrong, good and bad.

nurse prescribing: prescribing by a registered nurse who has been formally trained and registered with the NMC to prescribe medicines from a formulary.

parenteral route: non-gastrointestinal tract administrative route, including intravenous, intramuscular, topical, inhalants, subcutaneous and transdermal patches.

paternalism: believing that you know what is right for someone else, and excluding them from decision making.

Patient Medicines Administration Chart: commonly termed the patient's prescription chart. It should include all the necessary information of the prescribed medicine including the name of the medicine, the dose, the route and the frequency to enable the nurse to administer the medicine. The full patient details should be included. Local trust policy influences other aspects of the prescription chart including permissible abbreviations and alterations to prescriptions.

peer review: evaluation of a person's work or performance by a group of people in the same occupation, profession or industry.

per cent: means out of one hundred, and a percentage shows how many parts out of 100 we have. The symbol % is used to signify per cent. For example, 60% means we have 60 out of 100 parts. If a student scores 75 per cent in an examination, they have proportionally answered 75 out of every 100 questions correctly.

PEG tube: percutaneous endoscopic gastrostomy tube – a tube that is inserted by a surgeon through the wall of the abdomen into the stomach or jejunum to provide a way of administering nutrition to patients who have been assessed as having swallowing difficulties. In some cases is used as a means of administering nutrition if a person requires supplementary food.

peripheral cannula: a short hollow tube that is inserted into a superficial vein, usually in the hand or arm.

pharmacist: a pharmacy degree-qualified person in the community, hospital or pharmaceutical industry. They can check all aspects of prescriptions, provide advice on both medicines and healthy lifestyle choices, and can manage pharmacy technicians and pharmacy support workers. In a hospital setting they can specialise in a particular discipline such as renal, liver or cancer therapies and participate in team meetings.

pharmacodynamics: the effect that the drug has on the body – in other words, how the drug works to achieve the expected effect.

pharmacology: derived from the Greek words *pharmakon* meaning 'drug' and *ology* meaning 'knowledge or study of'.

pharmacokinetics: looks at how the body affects a drug, relating to the body's ability to absorb a drug, to the body's ability to then distribute the drug to the site of action, and also to the metabolic processes required to make the drug suitable for elimination once it has had its effect.

placebo: a substance that has no pharmacological or therapeutic property, used to overcome the possible suggestive effect of the alternative intervention.

primary evidence: information gained directly from an investigation at the time it was studied, usually by the researcher undertaking the study.

procurement: the purchasing of goods and/or services at the best possible cost in the right quality and quantity, at the right time, in the right place and from the right source for the direct benefit or use of individuals such as patients in the case of the NHS.

qualitative research: a method of inquiry that aims to gather an in-depth understanding of human behaviour and experiences, and involves the interpretation of meaning.

quantitative research: the systematic investigation that involves collection and examination of numerical data.

quantum: the amount of monetary compensation awarded for a claim.

randomised controlled trial: an experimental design that involves random allocation of participants, either to an experimental group that receives some form of treatment or intervention, or to a control group that receives no special treatment or intervention.

ratio: the relationship between two quantities, or how much of one there is compared to another.

recruits: people enlisted onto a research projects.

reliability: the extent to which a research project or method would produce the same results if used on different occasions with the same object of study.

royal assent: the final stage for an Act of Parliament to become law.

secondary evidence: evidence that has been reproduced and interpreted from the original source.

side effects: unwanted symptoms that arise due to the drug having an effect on other areas of the body.

statins: drugs designed to reduce cholesterol levels in the blood. The medicines work by reducing the amount of cholesterol the liver makes so the body has to use the cholesterol that is already available, so reducing the overall amount of cholesterol in the blood.

statistical significance: refers to the probability that a particular result of a statistical test could be due to chance factors alone.

statute: a law enacted by Parliament, also known as a piece of primary legislation.

statutory instrument: a form of subordinate law.

subcutaneous: administration of a drug into the fatty tissue of the skin.

sublingually: under the tongue.

supplementary prescribing: part of a voluntary partnership between an independent prescriber (a doctor or dentist) and a supplementary prescriber to implement an agreed patient-specific Clinical Management Plan with the patient's agreement (DH).

suspensions: a medicine composed of fine particles of drug within a liquid. The solids do not dissolve in the liquid so separate on storage. Thorough shaking of a suspension is required before administration to ensure the drug is equally dispersed throughout the liquid.

sustained release: oral preparation specifically designed to take a longer time to digest and be absorbed so fewer doses are required in a day.

systematic review: a summary of research that uses explicit methods to perform a thorough literature search and critical appraisal of individual studies, usually randomised control trials, to identify the valid and applicable evidence.

teleological theory: an ethical theory where the consequences of an action define whether it is ethical.

therapeutic index: the range of dosages of a medicine that can achieve the therapeutic effect but not a toxic effect. Medicines with a narrow therapeutic index have only a small range of doses available to give a therapeutic effect after which they can become potentially lethal. Some medicines have a wide therapeutic index so there is a much more extensive choice of doses suitable for the patients.

tort: a civil wrong.

trespass to the person: intrusion to a person's property or person.

utilitarianism: an approach that considers the best action is the one that promotes the greatest utilty for the greatest number.

validity: the degree to which what is observed or measured is the same as what was purported to be observed or measured.

value: a rule that allows us to decide what is right and wrong.

variable: a factor in the research that may be liable to vary or change.

venepuncture: the procedure of inserting a needle into a vein. It can be used for obtaining samples of blood for analysis.

ventrogluteal: the site that uses the gluteus medius muscle of the hip for intramuscular injections.

veracity: accurate transmission of information.

vicarious liability: the liability of an employer when the employee commits a wrong while in their employment.

Volenti Non Fit Injuria: where risk is accepted then the person cannot be harmed.

voluntary manslaughter: where the defendant had the *mens rea* to carry out the act.

References

Abd-el-Maeboud KH. el-Nuggar,T, el-Hawi, EM, Mahmoud, SA and Abd-el-Hay, S. (1991) Rectal suppository commonsense and mode of insertion. *The Lancet*, 338: 798–800.

Alderson, P. and Groves, T. (2004) What doesn't work and how to show it? *British Medical Journal*, 328. 473.

Andreescu, C, Benoit, H, Mulsant, B and Emanuel, J (2008) Complementary and alternative medicine in the treatment of bipolar disorder – a review of the evidence. *Journal of Affective Disorders* 110: 16–26.

Asthma UK (2010) *Spacers*. Available online at: www.asthma.org.uk/all_about_asthma/medicines_treatments/spacers.html (accessed 21 March 2010).

Audit Commission (2001) *A spoonful of sugar – medicines management in the NHS*. London: Audit Commission.

Barron, C and Cocoman, A (2008) Administering intramuscular injections to children: what does the evidence say? *Journal of Children's and Young People's Nursing*, 2: 138–44.

BBC (2004) *Thalidomide – a second chance*, TV programme transcript. Available online at: www.bbc.co.uk/science/horizon/2004/thalidomidetrans.shtml (accessed 6 January 2010).

Beauchamp, TL and Childress, JF (2009) *Principles of biomedical ethics*, 6th edition. New York, Oxford: Oxford University Press.

Bendick, J (2009) *Galen and the gateway to medicine*. Bathgate ND: Ignatius Press.

Bergkvist, K., and Wengstrom, Y (2006) Symptom experiences during chemotherapy treatment – with focus on nausea and vomiting. *European Journal of Oncology Nursing*, 10: 21–9.

BHF (British Heart Foundation) (2009) Life-Saving Science reports on recent discoveries. Available online at www.bhf.org.uk (accessed 30 March 2010).

Bisset, N (1991) One man's poison, another man's medicine? *Journal of Ethnopharmacology*, 32: 71–81.

BNF (2010) *British National Formulary*, 59th ed. London: British Medical Association and Royal Pharmaceutical Society of Great Britain. Available online at: www.bnf.org.

BTS (British Thoracic Society) (2008) *Emergency Oxygen Use in Adult Patients*, Appendix 6. Available online at: www.brit-thoracic.org.uk/clinical-information/emergency-oxygen/emergency-oxygen-use-in-adult-patients.aspx (accessed 22 April 2010).

Carter, S and Taylor, D (2005) *A question of choice: Compliance in medicine taking*, 3rd edition. London: Medicines Partnership. Available online at: http://www.keele.ac.uk/pharmacy/npcplus/medicinespartnershipprogramme/medicinespartnershipprogrammepublications/aquestionofchoicecomplianceinmedicinetakin/research-qoc-compliance.pdf (accessed 20 May 2009).

Chowdhury, S (2006) Exploring the science of laxatives: mechanism and modes of action. *Nurse Prescribing*, 4 (3): 107–112.

Claxton, AJ, Cramer, J and Pierce, C (2001) A systematic review of the associations between dose regimes and medication compliance. *Clinical Therapeutics*, 23: 1296–310.

Clothier Report (1994) *Independent inquiry relating to deaths and injuries on the children's ward at Grantham and Kesteven General Hospital*. London: HMSO.

Connell, P, McKevitt, C and Wolfe, C (2005) Strategies to manage hypertension: a qualitative study with black Caribbean patients. *British Journal of General Practice*, 55: 357–61.

Davies, H (2003) The licensing of medicines, an overview of the licensing process as it applies to medicinal products in the UK, UKMi. Available online at: www.ukmi.nhs.uk/Med_info/licensing_process.pdf (accessed 11 March 2010).

De Pasquale, A (1984) Pharmacognosy: the oldest modern science. *Journal of Ethnopharmacology*, 11: 1–16.

Diabetes UK (2009) *Annual review checklist*. Available online at: www.diabetes.org.uk/MyLife-YoungAdults/Treatment-and-care/What-care-to-expect/Annual-reviews/ (accessed 28 January 2010).

DH (Department of Health (1997) *The New NHS Modern, Dependable*. London: DH.

DH (2001) *The expert patient: a new approach to chronic disease management for the 21st century*. London: DH.

DH (2003a) *Supplementary prescribing by nurses and pharmacists within the NHS in England: a guide for implementation*. Available online at: www.dh.gov.uk/prod_consum_dh/groups/dh_digitalassets/@dh/@en/documents/digitalasset/dh_4068431.pdf (accessed 29 March 2010).

DH (2003b) *Essence of care: patient focused benchmarks for clinical governance*. London: The Stationery Office.

DH (2004) *Building a safer NHS for patients: improving medication safety*. London: DH.

DH (2006a) *Modernising nursing careers: setting the direction*. London: The Stationery Office.

DH (2006b) *Our health, our care, our say: a new direction for community services*. London: The Stationery Office.

DH (2006c) *Improving patients' access to medicines: a guide to implementing nurse and pharmacist independent prescribing within the NHS in England*. Available at: www.dh.gov.uk/prod_consum_dh/groups/dh_digitalassets/@dh/@en/documents/digitalasset/dh_4133747.pdf (accessed 29 March 2010).

DH (2009) *Extending professional and occupational regulation*. The Report of the Working Group on Extending Professional Regulation. Available online at: www.dh.gov.uk/prod_consum_dh/groups/dh_digitalassets/documents/digitalasset/dh_102818.pdf (accessed 2 June 2010).

Dougherty, L and Lister, S (2008) *Royal Marsden Hospital manual of clinical nursing procedures*. Oxford: Wiley Blackwell.

Evans, D (2003) Hierarchy of evidence: a framework for ranking of evidence evaluating healthcare interventions. *Journal of Clinical Nursing*. 12: 77–84.

Galbraith, A, Bullock, S, Manias, E, Hunt, B and Richards, A (2007) *Fundamentals of pharmacology; an applied approach for nurses and health*. Harlow: Pearson Education.

Gert, B (2004) Definition of morality. Available online at: http://plato.stanford.edu/entries/morality-definition/ (accessed 4 January 2010).

Gillon R (1986) *Philosophical medical ethics*. London: John Wiley.

Gillon, R (2003) Ethics needs principles – four can encompass the rest – and respect for autonomy should be 'first among equals.' *Journal of Medical Ethics*, 29: 307–12.

Griffith, R (2006) Adverse drug reactions and non-compliance with prescribed medication. *Nurse Prescribing* 4 (2).

Griffiths, R, Griffiths, H and Jordan, S (2003) Administration of medicines part 1: The law and nursing. *Nursing Standard*. 18 (2): 47–53.

Guyatt, GH, Oxman, AD, Vist, G, Kunz, R, Falck-Ytter, Y, Alonso-Coello, P and Schünemann, HJ (2008) Rating quality of evidence and strength of recommendations GRADE: an emerging consensus on rating quality of evidence and strength of recommendations. *British Medical Journal*, 336: 924–26.

Heinrich, M (2000) Ethnobotany and its role in drug development. *Phytotherapy Research*, 14: 479–88.

Heyneman, CA (2003) Preoperative considerations: which herbal products should be discontinued before surgery? *Critical Care Nurse*, 23: 116–24.

Horne, R, Frost, S, Weinman, J, Wright, SM, Graupner, L and Hankins, M (2004) Medicine in a multicultural society: the effect of cultural background on beliefs about medications. *Social Science and Medicine*, 59: 1307–13.

Hoyles, C, Noss, R and Pozzi, S (2001) Proportional reasoning in nursing practice. *Journal for Research in Mathematics Education*, 32 (1): 4–27.

Jukes, L and Gilchrist, M (2006) Concerns about numeracy skills of nursing students. *Nurse Education in Practice* 6: 192–8.

Kelly, J, D'Cruz, G and Wright, D (2009) A qualitative study of the problems surrounding medicine administration to patients with dysphagia. *Dysphagia*, 24: 49–56.

Kelly, LE and Colby, N (2003) Teaching medication calculation for conceptual understanding. *Journal of Nursing Education*, 42(10): 431–32.

King, KM and Rubin, G (2003) A history of diabetes: from antiquity to discovering insulin. *British Journal of Nursing*, 12: 1091–5.

Kozier, B, Erb, G, Berman, A, Snyder, S, Lake, R and Harvey, S (2008) *Fundamentals of nursing: concepts, process and practice*. Harlow: Pearson Education.

Leathard, A (2003) *Inter-professional collaboration: from policy to practice in health and social care*. Hove: Brunner-Routledge.

Lo, B (2006) HPV vaccine and adolescents' sexual activity. *British Medical Journal* 332: 1106–7.

Mantle, F and Tiran, D (2009) *An A–Z of complementary therapies for health professionals*. Edinburgh: Elsevier Science.

McKenry, I and Salerno, E. (1998) *Pharmacology in Nursing*, 20th edition. St Louis MO: Mosby.

MHRA (Medicines and Healthcare products Regulatory Agency) (2007) European Union Directive 2001/83, as cited in *A guide to what is a medicinal product*. London: HMSO.

MHRA (2004) *Reusable nebulisers*. Available online at: www.mhra.gov.uk/Publications/ Safetywarnings/MedicalDeviceAlerts/CON008559?useSecondary=&showpage=1 (accessed 4 June 2010).

MHRA (2008a) *Hyperiforce St John's Wort tablets*. Available online at: www.mhra.gov. uk/home/groups/pl-a/documents/websiteresources/con020730.pdf (accessed 28 January 2010).

MHRA (2008b) *Public health risk with herbal medicines: an overview*. Available online at: www.mhra.gov.uk/Safetyinformation/Generalsafetyinformationandadvice/ Adviceandinformationforconsumers/Usingherbalmedicines/index.htm (accessed 28 January 2010).

MHRA (2009) *Medicines and medical devices regulation: what you need to know?* London: MHRA.

Milton, JC, Hill-Smith, I and Jackson, SHD (2008) Prescribing for older people. *British Journal of Medicine*, 336: 606–9.

Montgomery J. (2003) *Health care law*. 2nd edition. New York: Oxford University Press.

National Collaborating Centre for Primary Care (2009) *Medicines adherence: involving patients in decisions about prescribed medicines and supporting adherence*. London: Royal College of General Practitioners.

NCCSDO (National Co-ordinating Centre for NHS Service and Delivery and Organisation Research and Development) (2005) *Concordance, adherence and compliance in medicine taking*. Available online at: www.medslearning.leeds.ac.uk/pages/documents/useful_docs/76-final-report%5B1%5D.pdf.

NHSIII (National Health Service Institution for Innovation and Improvement) (2005) The little bag that's big on savings: case study: Nottingham City Hospital. Available online at: www.institute.nhs.uk/resources/nhslive/3871/NHS%20LIVE%20Case%20Studies%20The%20Little%20bag.pdf (accessed 8 April 2010).

NHSIII (National Health Service Institute for Innovation and Improvement) (2008) *The productive ward: releasing time to care*. London: Institutes NHS.

NHSIII (2009) *Clinical medication review service*. Available online at: www.institute.nhs.uk/index.php?option=com_mtree&task=viewlink&link_id=4626&Itemid=4932#details (accessed 8 April 2010).

NICE (National Institute for Health and Clinical Excellence) (2003) *Management of chronic heart failure in primary and secondary care*. London: NICE.

NICE (2004) *The epilepsies: the diagnosis and management of epilepsies in adults and children in primary and secondary care*. London: NICE.

NICE (2006a) *Appraising orphan drugs*. Draft V3. Available online at www.nice.org.uk/niceMedia/pdf/smt/120705item4.pdf (accessed 15 March 2010).

NICE (2006b) *Moving beyond effectiveness in evidence synthesis: methodological issues in the synthesis of diverse sources of evidence*. London: NICE.

NMC (Nursing and Midwifery Council) (2007) *Standards for medicines management*. London: NMC.

NMC (2008) *The Code: standards of conduct, performance and ethics for nurses and midwives*. London: NMC.

NMC (2009) *Guidance on professional conduct for nursing and midwifery students*. London: NMC.

NPC (National Prescribing Centre) (2009a) *A guide to good practice in management of controlled drugs in primary care, England*, 3rd edition. Liverpool: The National Prescribing Centre.

NPC (2009b) *Business plan 2009–2010*. Liverpool: The National Prescribing Centre.

NPCRDC (National Primary Care Research and Development Centre) (2006) *The national evaluation of the pilot phase of the Expert Patient Programme – final report*. London: Department of Health.

NPSA (National Patient Safety Agency) (2005) *Wristbands for hospital inpatients improves safety*, Safer practice notice. London: NPSA.

NPSA (2007) *Standardising wristbands improves patient safety*, Safer practice notice. London: NPSA.

NPSA (2008) *Risk to patient safety of not using the NHS number as the national identifier for all patients*, Safer practice notice. London: NPSA.

NPSA (2009a) *NHS number: risk to patient safety of not using the NHS number as the national identifier for all patients*, Clarification statement. London: NPSA.

NPSA (2009b) *Safety in doses: improving the use of medicines in the NHS*. London: NPSA.

NPSA (2010) *Rapid response report NPSA/2010/RRR009: reducing harm from omitted and delayed medicines in hospital.* London: NPSA.

Odeh-Ramadan, RM and Remington, TL in Edwards, NM, Maurer, MS and Wellner, RB (eds) (2002) *Aging, heart disease and its management: facts and controversies.* Totowa NJ: Humana Press.

Page, C, Curtis, M, Sutter, M, Walker, M and Hoffman, B (2002) *Integrated pharmacology,* 2nd edition. Edinburgh: Mosby International.

Paracetamol Information Centre (2010) *Paracetamol in overdose.* Available online at: www.pharmweb.net/pwmirror/pwy/paracetamol/pharmwebpic9.html (accessed 17 January 2010).

Parnés, A and Lagan, KM (2007) Larval therapy in wound management: a review. *International Journal of Clinical Practice,* 61 (3): 488–93.

Pocock, SJ (2004) *Clinical trials: a practical approach.* New York: John Wiley & Sons.

Proulx, N, Fréchette, D, Toye, B, Chan, J and Kravcik, S (2005) Delays in the administration of antibiotics are associated with mortality from adult acute bacterial meningitis. *Qualitative Journal of Medicine,* 98 (4): 291–8.

Public Health Resource Unit (1999) *Critical appraisal skills programme.* Available online at: www.phru.nhs.uk/Pages/PHD/CASP.htm (accessed 8 April 2010).

RCGP (Royal College of General Practitioners) (2009) *Medicines adherence: involving patients in decisions about prescribed medicines and supporting adherence.* London: RCGP.

RPSGB (Royal Pharmaceutical Society of Great Britain) (2007) *Code of Ethics for Pharmacists and Pharmacy Technicians.* Available online at: www.rpsgb.org.uk/pdfs/coeppt.pdf (accessed 30 March 2010).

Sackett, DL, Rosenberg, WM, Gray, JA, Haynes, RB and Richardson, WS (1996) Evidence based medicine: what it is and what it isn't. *British Medical Journal,* 312 (7023): 71–2.

Schier, JG, Howland, MA, Hoffman, RS and Nelson, LS (2003) Fatality from administration of labetalol and crushed extended release nifedipine. *The Annals of Pharmacotherapy,* 37 (10): 1420–3.

Schwartz, L, Preece, PE and Hendry, RA (2002) *Medical ethics: a case based approach.* Edinburgh, London, New York: Saunders.

Sharma, P and Singh, G (2002) A review of plant species used to treat conjunctivitis. *Phytotherapy Research,* 16: 1–22.

Spear, BB, Heath-Chiozzi, M and Huff, J (2001) Clinical application of pharmacogenetics. *Trends in Molecular Medicine,* 7: 201–4.

Steenvoorde, P, Jacobi, CE, Van Doorn, L and Oskam, J (2007) Maggot debridement therapy of infected ulcers: patient and wound factors influencing outcome: a study on 101 patients with 117 wounds. *Annals The Royal College of Surgeons of England,* 89 (6): 596–602.

Stokes, P (2009) Pensioner 'unlawfully killed' by nurse's insulin overdose. *The Telegraph.* Available online at: www.telegraph.co.uk/news/uknews/5061193/Pensioner-unlawfully-killed-by-nurses-insulin-overdose.html (accessed 1 April 2010).

Thomas, A and Young, S (2008) An introduction to pharmacodynamics. *Practice Nursing,* 19: 596–600.

Thompson, IE, Melia, KM and Boyd, KM (2001) *Nursing Ethics,* 4th edition. Oxford: Churchill Livingstone.

Townsley, CA, Selby, R and Siu, LL (2005) Systematic reviews of barriers to the recruitment of older patients with cancer onto clinical trials. *Journal of Clinical Oncology,* 23 (13): 3112–24.

Walsh, M and Ford, P (1989) *Nursing rituals: research and rational actions.* Oxford: Butterworth–Heinemann.

Watson, R (2000) Medications and older people. *Nursing Older People*, 12 (6): 21–5.

Weeks, KW, Lyne, P and Torrance, C (2000) Written drug dose errors made by students: the threat to clinical effectiveness and the need for a new approach. *Clinical Effectiveness in Nursing* 4 (1): 20–9.

WHO (World Health Organisation) (2003) *Adherence to long term therapies: evidence for action.* Geneva: WHO.

WHO (2009) *Medicines Strategy and Policies: WHO Drug Information Vol 23, No 3.* Available online at: www.who.int/druginformation (accessed December 2009).

Wright, K. (2006) Student nurses need more than maths to improve their drug calculations skills. *Nurse Education Today*, 27 (4): 278–85.

Wright, K. (2007) Student nurses need more than maths to improve their drug calculating skills. *Nurse Education Today*, 27 (4): 278–85.

Wright, K. (2008a) Drug calculations part 1: a critique of the formula used by nurses. *Nursing Standard*, 22 (36): 40–2.

Wright, K (2008b) Drug calculations part 2: alternative strategies to the formula. *Nursing Standard*, 22 (37): 42–4.

Index